Familial Cancer Management

Edited by
Walter Weber
Associate Professor of Medical Oncology University of Basel
Basel, Switzerland
and
Scientific Secretary
Swiss Cancer League
Bern, Switzerland

John J. Mulvihill
Graduate School of Public Health
Department of Human Genetics
University of Pittsburgh
Pittsburgh, Pennsylvania

Steven A. Narod
Department of Medicine
Division of Medical Genetics
Montreal General Hospital
Montreal, Canada

CRC Press
Boca Raton   New York   London   Tokyo

Library of Congress Cataloging-in-Publication Data

Familial cancer management / edited by Walter Weber, John J. Mulvihill, and
  Steven A. Narod.
        p.   cm.
    Includes bibliographical references and index.
    ISBN 0-8493-4782-3 (alk. paper)
    1. 1. Cancer—Genetic aspects. 2. Cancer—Epidemiology. 3. Genetic counseling.
  4. Cancer—Chemoprevention. I. Weber, W. (Walter) II. Mulvihill, John J., 1943–
  III. Narod, Steven A..
    [DNLM: 1. Neoplasms—genetics. 2. Neoplasms—diagnosis. 3. Neoplasms—
  prevention & control. QZ 202 F1985 1996]
  RC268.4.F35   1996
  616.99'4042—dc20
  DNLM/DLC
  for Library of Congress   95-31247
                                                                                                CIP

© 1996 by CRC Press, Inc.

No claim to original U.S. Government works
International Standard Book Number 0-8493-4782-3/96
Library of Congress Card Number 95-31247
Printed in the United States of America   2 3 4 5 6 7 8 9 0
Printed on acid-free paper

DEDICATION

This book is dedicated to Lemuel Herrara, M.D., an astute clinician who first described an interstitial deletion of chromosome 5q in 1986, leading to the detection of the adenomatous polyposis coli (APC) gene. Lemuel encouraged us in editing this book and initiated chapter 8 on the surgical management of familial cancer syndromes. At the second UICC strategy meeting on familial cancer management in Woods Hole, he stressed the importance of practical guidance of physicians worldwide. Lemuel passed away too early in May 1995.

PREFACE

Every human trait clusters in families. This is also true for cancer. Familial clustering of cancer is well known from epidemiologic studies. This can be due to chance, shared environmental influences, shared genes, and chance-environmental-gene-interaction. Family studies are a key to the understanding of the environmental and genetic etiology of chronic disease. Cancer families are human models of susceptibility to neoplasia. There are now blood tests available to help identify which persons do and which do not carry characteristics predisposing them to cancer. Hereditary metabolic variations affecting the metabolism of carcinogens can be identified.

More and more people are aware of, and anxious about their cancer risk. High-risk individuals can benefit from screening programs. Intervention trials can be initiated. In medical practice, the patient workup should include a carefully obtained family history. This simple method has the potential for reduction of cancer morbidity and mortality. It is therefore surprising that this part of the patient workup is frequently given little attention in clinical practice. Every person should create his or her own family tree and discuss it with his/her own doctor. This is a step everybody can take to improve their health. This book is a guide for making the best possible use of the family history for cancer control.

THE EDITORS

Dr. Walter Weber is medical oncologist in private practice in Basel, Switzerland. He is Privatdozent (associate professor) for medical oncology at the University of Basel and Scientific secretary of the Swiss Cancer League. He is a graduate of the University of Basel (M.D., 1969). He trained for general internal medicine in the U.S., then for hematology and oncology in the Basel University Hospital. He obtained the European Certification on Medical Oncology (1989). His research interests are in prevention and treatment of gastrointestinal cancer and in exploring the family history for cancer control. He is in charge of research funding in the Swiss Cancer League and coordinates the UICC Familial Cancer Project.

Dr. John J. Mulvihill is a pediatrician, medical geneticist, and epidemiologist with 20 years of experience at the National Cancer Institute. In addition, he was Director of the Interinstitute Medical Genetics Program. In 1990, he became founder, chair, and professor of Human Genetics at the University of Pittsburgh and co-director of the Pittsburgh Genetics Institute. He is also Professor of Pediatrics and of Molecular Genetics and Biochemistry. A graduate of the College of the Holy Cross, Dartmouth Medical School, and the University of Washington, he was on the house staffs of the University of Washington and Johns Hopkins Hospitals. Dr. Mulvihill is a member of ten professional societies as well as co-founder and second president of the International Genetic Epidemiology Society. In addition to belonging to the editorial boards of six scientific journals, he is coeditor-in-chief of the journal *Genetic Epidemiology*. Dr. Mulvihill's research has focused on the genetics of human cancer, with emphasis on hereditary and familial factors, and on reproduction by cancer survivors. He spearheads interdisciplinary epidemiologic, clinical, and laboratory studies aimed at finding the single gene that predispose to cancer and at searching for possible genetic damage following intensive cancer treatment.

Dr. Steven A. Narod is Chair of Breast Cancer Research, University of Toronto at Women's College Hospital, Toronto, Ontario. Beforehand, he was professor of medicine at the Division of Medical Genetics of Royal Victoria Hospital and Montreal General Hospital in Montreal, Quebec. He is a graduate of the University of British Columbia in Vancouver (M.D., 1979). He trained in community medicine at the University of Ottawa and in medical genetics at the Hospital for Sick Children in Toronto. He was a fellow in cancer epidemiology in the program on viral and hereditary factors in carcinogenesis, Unit of Mechanisms of Carcinogenesis, at the WHO International Agency for Research on Cancer in Lyons, France from 1988 until 1990. His research interests are in mutation epidemiology, reproductive epidemiology, linkage and mapping, screening for cancer, cancer family syndromes including multiple endocrine neoplasia, and hereditary breast cancer.

CONTRIBUTORS

Sean Davis, B.S.E.
Graduate School of Public Health
Department of Human Genetics
University of Pittsburgh
Pittsburgh, Pennsylvania

Kenneth R. Fromkin, M.D.
School of Medicine
Yale University
New Haven, Connecticut

Raanan Gillon, F.R.C.P.
General Medical Practitioner
Professor of Medical Ethics
Imperial College of Science,
  Technology, and Medicine
London University
London, United Kingdom

Ophira Ginsburg, M.Sc.
Division of Medical Genetics
Department of Medicine
McGill University
Montreal, Canada

Brian K. Hart, B.S.Ed.
Graduate School of Public Health
Department of Human Genetics
University of Pittsburgh
Pittsburgh, Pennsylvania

Lemuel Herrera, M.D.*
Chief of Surgical Oncology
Health Science Center
Department of Surgery
Brooklyn, New York

Lennart Iselius, M.D.
Department of Surgery
Karolinska Hospital
Stockholm, Sweden

Patrick M. Lynch, M.D.
Department of Gastrointestinal
  Oncology and Digestive Diseases
M.D. Anderson Cancer Center
Texas Medical Center
Houston, Texas

Solange D. MacArthur, M.D.
Assistant Professor of Surgery
State University of New York
Health Science Center
Brooklyn, New York

David Malkin, M.D.
Assistant Professor
Divisions of Oncology and
  Immunology and Cancer Research
Department of Pediatrics
The Hospital for Sick Children
University of Toronto
Toronto, Ontario, Canada

Jukka-Pekka Mecklin, M.D.
Assistant Professor of Surgery
Jyvaskyla Central Hospital
Jyvaskyla, Finland

Hansjakob Müller, M.D.
Head
Department of Medical Genetics
University Children's Hospital, and
Department of Research
University Hospital
Basel, Switzerland

John J. Mulvihill, M.D.
Graduate School of Public Health
Department of Human Genetics
University of Pittsburgh
Pittsburgh, Pennsylvania

Steven A. Narod, M.D.[**]
Department of Medicine
Division of Medical Genetics
Montreal General Hospital
Montreal, Quebec, Canada

Rodney J. Scott, Ph.D.
Human Genetics Research Group
University Hospital
Basel, Switzerland

Maria Shaffer-Gordon, M.S.
Graduate School of Public Health
Department of Human Genetics
University of Pittsburgh
Pittsburgh, Pennsylvania

Hans-Rudolf Stoll, R.N., M.Sc.
Spitalexterne Onkologiepflege
Basel, Switzerland

Grant N. Stemmermann, M.D.
Medical Center
Department of Pathology and
  Laboratory Medicine
University of Cincinnati
Cincinnati, Ohio

Walter Weber, M.D.
Medical Oncology
Scientific Secretary
Swiss Cancer League
Bern, Switzerland

Nils Wilking, M.D.
Department of Oncology
Radiumhemmet
Karolinska Hospital
Stockholm, Sweden

[*] Deceased
[**] Dr. Narod has recently tranferred to the University of Toronto in Toronto, Ontario where he serves as Chair of Breast Cancer Research at Women's College Hospital

TABLE OF CONTENTS

Chapter 1

MOLECULAR BIOLOGY OF CANCER INDUCTION, TUMOR SUPPRESSION, AND GROWTH PROMOTION

Rodney J. Scott

CONTENTS

I. INTRODUCTION

There are many facets to the development of cancer that singularly are not likely to initiate a cell along the path towards malignancy. Only when all the events that give rise to a committed neoplastic cell have accumulated does a malignancy occur that eventually leads to invasion and metastasis. The circumstances that underlie the change from normality to malignancy do not necessarily have to occur in any given order; it appears only to be the number that is important. This applies both for sporadic and familial forms of cancer. In this review the mechanisms of induction of disease shall be discussed with respect to familial cancer, followed by the immediate events thereafter pertaining to tumor suppression and growth promotion. A major difference between sporadic cancer and its familial counterpart is that one of the events involved in the "cascade of calamity" leading to the development of disease is already present, therefore, only n–1 events (where n = the hypothetical number of events leading to the formation of sporadic disease) are necessary for disease development.

1

II. CANCER INDUCTION

It is estimated that persons coming from families where there is a well-defined cancer family syndrome represent approximately 0.1% of all cancer cases; however, between 5 and 10% of all cancers may be associated with a hereditary predisposition of one form or another.[1] As this encompasses virtually all cancer types, the total number of cases therefore represents many different ways in which disease can develop in persons susceptible to neoplasia. Not only can direct genetic traits be observed; it is also becoming increasingly evident that ecogenetic traits are important in disease development. Persons having a genetic predisposition towards cancer development are not born with the disease, but have the propensity to develop cancer given the appropriate environment.

A well-studied example of an ecogenetic trait is that of bladder cancer. Epidemiological studies have shown that this disease is associated with smoking and occupational exposure to various arylamines,[2,3] however not all smokers or chemical workers develop bladder cancer. In addition, there exist familial aggregations of bladder cancer, implying an autosomal dominant mode of inheritance.[4] Molecular investigations into such families have revealed that there appears to be no direct link between a tumor suppressor gene or oncogene to this disease. There is, however, a very strong correlation between a person's ability to metabolize aromatic amines (through the acetylation pathway) that are present in the environment[5] and the development of bladder cancer — such that slow acetylators appear to be predisposed to the development of bladder cancer, whereas rapid acetylators tend not to develop disease even when they are exposed to the same environmental stress. Therefore, in this particular example the ability to rapidly convert a particular carcinogen into an inactive compound is missing, which predisposes persons to the development of bladder cancer.[2] It can therefore be concluded that a person does not necessarily have the inherent ability to develop bladder cancer but given the right environmental conditions is capable of doing so. Should they never see the appropriate stimulus, they would be at no more risk of developing bladder cancer than persons who are rapid acetylators.[2]

Familial cancers associated with a confirmed genetic trait (i.e., an autosomal dominantly inherited disease predisposition) are by far the most intensively investigated diseases as the phenotype is more apparent and can be easily traced through a person's pedigree. A list of some of the more common familial cancer syndromes is given in Table 1. Cancer induction in familial cancer appears, on current evidence, to be no different to that observed in sporadic disease. The model for an inherited cancer susceptibility is that of retinoblastoma, where the familial predisposition to disease development is passed from generation to generation as a recessive trait; only if a somatic mutation in the remaining wild type allele occurs will the disease manifest itself,[6,7] with little difference between the two forms, inherited or sporadic, in regards to disease progression.

TABLE 1
Familial Cancer Syndromes and Their Corresponding Molecular Defect

Syndrome	Gene	Locus
Familial adenomatous polyposis	APC	5q21
Hereditary non-polyposis colorectal cancer	hMSH2	2p16
	hMLH	3p21
	PMS1	2q31-32
	PMS2	7p22
Familial breast cancer	BRCA1	17q21
	BRCA2	13q12-13
Familial atypical malignant mole and melanoma syndrome	MLM	9p21
Multiple endocrine neoplasia (type 1)	MEN1	11q13
Multiple endocrine neoplasia (type 2A)	RET	10q11
von Hippel-Lindau disease	g7	3p25
Neurofibromatosis 1	NF1	17q11
Neurofibromatosis 2	NF2	22q12
Li-Fraumeni syndrome	p53	17p13
Wilms tumor	WT1	11p13
Retinoblastoma	Rb1	13q14
Neuroblastoma	NB	1p36
Nevoid basal cell carcinoma syndrome	BCNS	9q31
Tuberous sclerosis 1	TCS1	9q34
Tuberous sclerosis 2	TCS2	16p13
Renal cell carcinoma	RCC	3q14
Beckwith-Wiedemann syndrome	BWS	11p15

As a general rule, familial cancer induction can be modeled around the concept of loss of heterozygosity (LOH) where one wild type allele and one mutated allele are inherited together. This in itself does not imply that disease will automatically occur. Only after the wild type allele has been lost will the characteristics of the particular disease begin to become apparent. The concept of LOH conforms with the multistage theory of cancer development (i.e., that of initiation, promotion, and progression), the mechanism of which can be explained in several ways. Recombination is one possible mechanism that could result in LOH. In cells that are heterozygous for a given gene on two homologous chromosomes, reciprocal recombination in the chromosome segment between the gene and the centromere can occur giving rise to a loss of one of the genes. Alternatively, gene conversion in the region of the marker gene can also occur, again leading to a loss of one of the genes.[8] Together, recombination and gene conversion represent two important ways by which dominantly inherited cancer susceptibilities are thought to transpire, so much so that at least 32 genetic entities have been described that are believed to be generated by one of these two mechanisms.[9] The following discussion on cancer induction in familial cancer is presented through several examples where genes or gene loci are known.

The elegant work of Fearon and Vogelstein in 1990 established that in colorectal cancer (CRC) the same genetic changes occur as in the rare familial adenomatous polyposis (FAP) syndrome and sporadic CRC.[10] The only difference between the two being the presence of a germline mutation in the Adenomatous Polyposis Coli (*APC*) gene. In comparing sporadic disease to corresponding familial forms, the major differences appear to be age of onset and likelihood of multifocal disease. However, not all cells in a susceptible tissue become malignant, implying that secondary events are required for disease development. Additional genetic changes occurring within susceptible tissue are not well understood, however, there appear to be different mechanisms that can initiate progression. The FAP syndrome is unusual in that there appear to be several explanations that can account for initiation of disease. Originally, it was proposed that FAP followed the model described for retinoblastoma (i.e., loss of heterozygosity), but as more mutations were recognized it became evident that LOH was not necessary for adenoma formation.[11] Gene dosage is an alternative effect that may be operating in FAP; as only one copy of the *APC* gene is functional, the amount that is required for correct physiological function is lacking, leading to an increase in crypt cell proliferation throughout the colon and rectum. There is evidence to show that polyp formation occurs after loss of the wild type allele.[12] As most mutations found to date result in either stop codons, frame shifts, or nonsense proteins, this model appears to be compatible.[13] Alternatively, development of disease in FAP could be associated with a somatic site-specific mutation within a background of elevated crypt cell proliferation, again leading to polyp formation.[14] In a recent review, Nagase and Nakamura have shown that the stochastic model of tumor development in FAP is the most likely,[13] additionally, our data confirm these findings with respect to polyp number and types of mutation found (not published). In summary, for FAP it appears that a germline mutation is sufficient for hyperplasia, corresponding to Knudson's "first hit", followed by a "second hit" that inactivates the wild type allele giving rise to polyp formation. Thereafter, additional events are necessary for adenocarcinoma development.

Other familial cancer syndromes have also been extensively studied, such as the Li-Fraumeni syndrome and the multiple endocrine neoplasias (1 and 2). The Li-Fraumeni syndrome is associated with germline mutations in the tumor suppressor gene p53, which has also been shown to be the most commonly mutated gene in human neoplastic disease.[15] In 1969, Li and Fraumeni defined this familial syndrome as having the following characteristics: an index patient with either sarcoma, breast cancer, brain tumor, leukemia, or adrenocortical carcinoma, under the age of 45 years, with other family members suffering from the same diseases occurring at any age.[16] Since this definition was proposed and the underlying genetic defect identified, many more characteristics can be included such as seminoma, adenocarcinoma, carcinoid, and histiocytoma.[17-21] Investigations into the mechanisms that occur within a given cell that leads to disease indicate that there is a loss of heterozygosity (LOH) at the *p53* locus. Before an understanding of the events that occur in persons predisposed to developing disease in this syndrome, a brief description of the function of the wild type gene is necessary. Many studies have now shown that wild type (wt) *p53* functions as a negative regulator of cell growth and that it may play a central role in genomic stability and DNA repair. The mechanism by which *p53* can effect the expression of certain critical genes within the cell cycle has been reported to be due to the binding of p53 to a specific DNA sequence that is associated with only a few genes such as GADD45 (Growth Arrest and DNA Delay), muscle creatine kinase, and the mdm2 (Mouse Double Minute) genes.[22,23] On examination, mutations in the p53 gene appear to be enigmatic in that different mutations give rise to products that have different functions. There can be a gain of function leading to new undesirable characteristics that would normally not be seen, or a loss of function that implies a lack of coordination within the cell (for a review see Harris and Hollstein).[15] Together, all the findings appear to indicate that *p53* plays a key role in cell regulation.

It was originally believed that the Li-Fraumeni phenotype was restricted to a site within the *p53* gene at codon 248.[18] Since this original observation, many more mutations have been found in the *p53* gene; however, they occur within discrete domains implying that there are several sites within the *p53* gene that are absolutely critical for its function as indicated in Figure 1. Not all Li-Fraumeni families appear to be linked to the *p53* gene even though the classical constellation of tumors is present. This indicates that either there are other genes involved which are not related to *p53*, or genes up- or downstream of p53 are affected which result in altered *p53* expression. Finally, due to the central role that *p53* appears to play in maintaining cell homeostasis, treatment of patients who have been shown to carry a constitutional *p53* mutation must be carefully considered. Chemotherapy, radiation therapy, or both may increase the risk of an iatrogenic second cancer due to a failure in cell cycle checkpoint control which would normally come into play after exposure to such agents.[15]

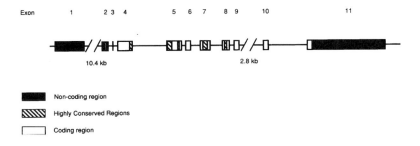

FIGURE 1. Schematic representation of the mutational "hot spots" found in the *p53* gene. The highly conserved regions are represented by diagonal stripes, which correspond to critical sites within the *p53* gene.

Hereditary non-polyposis colorectal cancer (HNPCC, previously known as the cancer family syndrome or Lynch syndromes I and II) possibly represents a new mechanism by which tumor development occurs within the colon. In 1993, two gene loci were defined that segregated with HNPCC which mapped to chromosome 2p and chromosome 3p, respectively.[24-26] It was observed that small di- and tri-nucleotide sequences were either amplified or reduced in length, indicating genomic instability probably occurring by a failure in mismatch repair.[27] Before the end of that year a gene had been localized on chromosome 2p that was shown to be mutated in a number of persons coming from families where an aggregation of non-polyposis colorectal cancer occurred.[27] The gene was identified based on the genetic properties that were observed in DNA isolated from tumors obtained from affected individuals. The finding that the genome was unstable indicated that a gene associated with either DNA synthesis or repair was involved. In comparing a yeast gene that performed a similar but not identical task (due to yeast not having di- or tri-nucleotide repeat sequences) Kolodner's group identified a human homolog.[28] Studies into HNPCC families revealed that this gene (termed *hMSH2*) segregated with affected persons and was therefore a strong candidate for an HNPCC gene. Further evidence was provided by Vogelstein's group, who proved independently that *hMSH2* was mutated in their collection of families.[29] The second locus that has been shown to be associated with the HNPCC phenotype harbors another DNA repair gene, termed *hMLH1*, which is also associated with microsatellite instability,[30,31] suggesting that mutations in any of the genes associated with mismatch repair may predispose to the HNPCC phenotype. Indeed, germline mutations in two other genes associated with mismatch repair have been reported in separate families termed *PMS1* and *PMS2*, respectively.[32] The two genes lie on chromosomes 2q31-32 and 7p22[32] and are expected to account for approximately 10% of all HNPCC families (R. Kolodner, personal communication).

The mechanisms by which a mutation in either the *hMSH2, hMLH1, PMS1,* or *PMS2* genes could give rise to colorectal tumors are not clearly understood; however, it is believed that during DNA replication slippage of the DNA polymerase occurs at di- or tri-nucleotide sequence chains that is not efficiently corrected by the repair enzyme encoded by the *hMSH2* gene.[28-31,33] The mechanism by which disease develops thereafter remains elusive, but is probably related to a change in the expression pattern of critical proteins associated with the cell cycle.[34] With respect to Knudson's "two hit" theory the initial event therefore remains the germline mutation in the *hMSH2* gene, followed presumably by LOH at the same locus (this, however, has not been observed to date for *hMSH2*); thereafter, due to the nature of the gene affected, the likelihood that errors occur at other sites within the genome is increased which may well account for further genetic changes seen later in tumor development.[29]

The disease first described by von Hippel and Lindau and named after them is characterized by the development of hemangioblastomas of the central nervous system and retina and renal cell carcinoma. The von Hippel-Lindau

(VHL) gene locus has been shown to lie on chromosome 3p25-3p36 and more recently a candidate gene has been found that lies within this region. From a genetic viewpoint, disease development can be modeled around Knudson's "two hit" theory,[35] as LOH has been observed in a large number of tumors coming from patients with this disease.[36,37] Investigations into the candidate gene (*g7*) have revealed substantial deletions in the VHL gene from persons with an inherited susceptibility to develop this disease.[36] The function of the gene is currently unknown but it is expressed in developing brain and kidney, and in adult brain, cerebellum, and prostate. The *g7* gene appears to represent yet another example of a tumor suppressor gene associated with a particular phenotype.

Multiple endocrine neoplasia represents another familial disease that is subdivided into four different types, MEN1, MEN2A, MEN2B, and familial medullary thyroid cancer (FMTC).

The three diseases MEN2A, MEN2B, and FMTC, can be defined as follows: MEN2A comprises families where there are persons affected with medullary thyroid cancer (MTC) with either pheochromocytoma or parathyroid disease; MEN2B contains persons with MTC with or without pheochromocytoma, other characteristic abnormalities, but without parathyroid cancer; and FMTC is defined as families where there is a minimum of four persons affected with MTC but no evidence of pheochromocytoma or parathyroid disease.

Genetic linkage studies of MEN2A and MTC families led to the identification of a locus on chromosome 10q11.2 encompassing the RET proto-oncogene.[39] Since the localization of the MEN2A and MTC locus, many patients with MEN2A have been studied and it was revealed that a high proportion of them contain mutations in the RET gene. The RET gene is a tyrosine kinase which contains two highly conserved cysteine residues in the extracellular domain of the protein.[38] Furthermore, the site of mutation may influence the phenotype; for instance, the proportion of mutations occurring at codon 634 of the RET gene is higher in MEN2A than FMTC suggesting that this mutation is related to the phenotype.[38] Evidence implies that MEN2B is not associated with the RET gene as no mutations have been found in affected persons coming from such families.[38]

In the case of MEN1 the mechanism by which disease develops is not clear. Originally it was thought to represent another example of a tumor suppressor gene that followed Knudson's "two hit" hypothesis as LOH was observed for markers on chromosome 11q in tumors coming from patients with MEN1.[40] Recently, however, a family has been reported where there exist two affected homozygotes and one heterozygote. Symptoms of the homozygotes are almost identical to those of the heterozygote who presumably develops disease via the mechanism of LOH; the only difference being that the homozygotes are sterile.[41] The finding that homozygotes appear not to be at any greater risk of disease development leaves open the question as to what role LOH plays in this disease and whether it requires a new interpretation of the "two hit" hypothesis. Several explanations are possible: in MEN1 tumors the second mutation is usually a deletion involving most of chromosome 11,[42,43] therefore the two mutations may be insufficient to entirely eliminate the function of the MEN1 gene, or loss of the MEN1 gene is not enough for tumor development. The likelihood that parental imprinting can account for such a situation is unlikely given that the disease is equally transmitted through both parents, although it is seen in hereditary paraganglioma where the disease gene must be inherited through the paternal allele.[44,45]

Breast cancer represents one of the leading causes of death in women today and as such attracts a large and growing number of studies into its cause. By far the most consistent finding is the increased risk of disease development in first degree relatives of breast cancer patients. This epidemiological finding is now being supported by recent discoveries of genes that appear to be associated with the development of breast cancer. In 1990 a locus on chromosome 17q was identified that appeared to predispose certain persons to the development of breast cancer;[46] further support was forthcoming in 1993 when the International Breast Cancer consortium reported its findings with respect to the 17q locus, providing indisputable proof that the 17q locus did indeed predispose to familial breast cancer.[47-49] The *BRCA1* locus appears to predispose women not only to breast cancer but also ovarian cancer, so much so that the BRCA1 gene should not be called a breast cancer susceptibility gene but rather an ovarian cancer susceptibility gene with breast cancer as a common complication, as a higher percentage of breast-ovarian cancer families segregated with the BRCA1 locus compared to breast cancer families alone (D.T. Bishop, personal communication). Recently, the *BRCA1* gene has been identified and it appears that is a tumor suppressor gene as allelic losses of chromosome 17q are a consistent finding in breast cancer tumors.[50,51,52] Furthermore, the gene has certain characteristics such as a C_3HC_4 zinc-finger domain and an excess of acidic residues, suggesting that it is a transcription factor.[51] A second predisposing gene *BRCA2* has been identified that maps to chromosome 13q12-13. Again, due to a high percentage of tumors showing allelic loss at this locus a tumor suppressor gene is suspected. Similar to *BRCA1*, *BRCA2* appears to confer a high risk of early onset breast cancer in women. In contrast to *BRCA1*, *BRCA2* may also contribute to male breast cancer susceptibility as several cases of male breast cancer were identified in linked families whereas none were observed in *BRCA1* linked families.[53]

In summary, tumor induction in familial cancer appears to occur via the mechanism of LOH. There are, however, indications that LOH may not be the only mechanism by which disease can develop in a susceptible person and that perhaps other mechanisms may be involved.

III. TUMOR SUPPRESSION

The initiation of cancer in persons who have inherited a genetic predisposition appears either to begin via the LOH pathway or they have inherited a genetic instability syndrome which predisposes these persons to replication errors that may lead to the development of disease. Additionally, mechanisms must exist within persons who are predisposed to the development of disease that prevent the vast majority of cells from becoming malignant.

There is a surfeit of evidence to show that there are genes capable of antagonizing tumor development. Cell fusion studies between tumor cells with one or more genetic changes and normal cells indicate that a normal complement of genes can revert a tumor phenotype back to a normal one.[54] Such evidence favors the idea that there are genes which can suppress the tumor phenotype. Since the pioneering work of Harris in 1969,[54] many tumor suppressor genes have been isolated which when transfected into tumors cells cause a reversion in phenotype.[55,56] Along with the growing number of tumor suppressor genes that have been isolated to date, there is ample evidence indicating that others exist as judged by LOH studies on tumor material. A list of some of the chromosomes affected in specific diseases is shown in Table 2.

Studies have consistently shown that the short arm of chromosome 11 contains within it at least two if not more tumor suppressor genes that can cause reversion when reinserted into tumor cells that have alterations in other tumor suppressor genes lying on other chromosomes.[57] This indicates that there is redundancy within normal cells such that genetic changes which lead to tumor development can be overridden via other unaffected genes. In the case of familial cancer this is clearly apparent as not all cells will develop into tumor cells. Returning to the disease of FAP, a sequence of events can be delineated that starts with a germline mutation in the APC gene followed by mutations in the MCC gene, ras oncogene, DCC gene, and the p53 gene,[58] thus providing indirect evidence that there are other tumor suppressor genes on other chromosomes which can, when present in their normal state, inhibit the development of disease.

One question that remains difficult to explain, especially in relation to familial cancers, is the specificity of the tumors that arise. In the Li-Fraumeni syndrome by far the commonest tumor within the spectrum is the soft tissue sarcoma which occurs in approximately 22% of all patients.[59] Interestingly, there is no evidence of an increased risk of developing colorectal cancer in predisposed persons. However, p53 mutations are a common event in the genesis of colorectal cancer. This observation may indicate two things:(1) p53 plays only a minor role in cell regulation within the colon, and (2) only when other tumor suppressive genes have been compromised will loss of p53 lead to the progression of adenoma to adenocarcinoma within the colon.[15] Similarly, HNPCC only presents with a defined spectrum of diseases, again implying that there are tissue-specific differences with respect to the function of any given gene associated with tumor suppression.

In summary, it appears that several tumor suppressor genes need to be inactivated prior to the establishment of neoplasia. Evidence comes from many

TABLE 2
Chromosome Losses Associated With Tumor
Progression in Different Human Cancers

Type of disease	Genetic change
Small cell lung carcinoma	3p loss 13q loss 17p loss
Colorectal cancer	5q loss 17p loss 18q loss
Osteosarcoma	13q loss 17p loss
Uterine cervical carcinoma	3p loss
Non-small cell lung carcinoma	3p loss 11p loss 13q loss 17p loss
Gastric carcinoma	1q loss 12q loss
Urinary bladder carcinoma	9q loss 11p loss 17p loss
Hepatocellular carcinoma	4 loss 16q loss HPV
Prostate carcinoma	10p loss 16q loss
Breast cancer	3p loss 13q loss 17p loss

From Yokota J. and Sugimura, T., *FASEB J.*, 7, 920, 1993.
With permission.

studies which reveal, if not directly, that there are putative tumor suppressor genes spread throughout the genome. Due to the apparent redundancy of tumor suppressor genes, it appears that more than one of them needs to be mutated before cells escape their normal regulatory controls.

IV. GROWTH PROMOTION

Taken together, the results of experimental models and those inferred from epidemiological studies of the age-dependent incidence of disease in humans indicate that there are between four and six independent events that need to occur before cancer develops.[60,61] This implies that in the situation where tumor suppressor genes are involved only two or three must be inactivated for tumor formation, as two independent genetic events are necessary for each tumor suppressor gene.[62,63] It should be remembered that most mutations result in cell death and that it is only relatively few that lead to uncontrolled cell growth. As the process of carcinogenesis can be subdivided into three stages — initiation, promotion, and progression — it can be assumed that initiation has already occurred in persons who have an inherited germline mutation which predisposes them to the development of disease. Promotion and progression occur thereafter and are characterized by somatic events which are similar to those seen in sporadic cancer. Presumably, the second event is loss of the remaining wild type allele which would then give those cells a selective growth advantage. Further somatic changes that involve other tumor suppressor genes or oncogenes may then occur.

Probably the best example of somatic changes that are associated with promotion and progression can be seen in the development of familial forms of colorectal cancer. Interestingly, the genetic changes that have been studied in familial colorectal cancer appear to be virtually identical to those seen in sporadic cases of the same disease; there are indications that this is also true for other types of neoplastic disease such as glioblastoma development.[64] Growth-promoting effects therefore appear to be associated with further LOH at other loci, implying that some event has occurred that results in genomic instability. Evidence of an increased genomic instability comes from studies on fibroblasts isolated from Li-Fraumeni syndrome patients as they quickly become aneuploid and acquire immortality *in vitro*.[65] Other studies centered around cells that are lacking *p53* indicate that they are unable to repair DNA damage efficiently. In addition, there is a tendency for these cells to show inappropriate amplification and recombinational events[56,66,67] and, as a consequence, defects in G1-S checkpoint control of the cell cycle[66] that lead to premature entry into S phase which eventuates in tetraploidy.[68] This type of instability is believed to favor the development of neoplasia as there is a general breakdown of control within the cell as more and more genetic changes accumulate. The disease of ataxia telangiectasia (AT) represents an interesting model with respect to genomic instability. Following ionizing radiation to normal cells AT gene(s) are expressed, the gene products of which interact with the tumor suppressor gene *p53*; elevated levels of *p53* lead to G1 arrest such that DNA repair can proceed prior to DNA synthesis and subsequent cell division.[34] In ataxia telangiectasia, however, the circumstances are somewhat different. After ionizing radiation there is no respite in replicative DNA synthesis, leading to the situation where a cell will have an increased likelihood of acquiring a heritable genetic abnormality that can be passed on to its daughter cells. Similarly, cells that lack *p53* also will not be able to trigger G1 arrest, again creating a situation where an increased genomic instability is observed. It is therefore not surprising that *p53* is one of the most commonly mutated genes thus far discovered in human cancer, and that persons who harbor p53 mutations tend in general to have a poorer prognosis than those who do not.

For specific forms of familial colorectal cancer, other mechanisms may be more likely. For example, the underlying defect that gives rise to HNPCC appears to offer an explanation as to why there is progression of tumor development once the disease is initiated. As the inherited predisposition is a defect in mismatch repair, failure to correct such a DNA error could conceivably knock out any given tumor suppressor or oncogene such that somatic changes occur quite rapidly thereafter.[29] Interestingly, the prognosis of persons who have inherited a germline mutation in their *hMSH2* gene, if caught early enough, appears to be very good, indicating that only when the activity of the *hMSH2* gene product is absent will there be a likelihood of tumor development.[29]

In summary, once a cell has acquired a particular growth advantage it appears that the likelihood of an additional change occurring is increased such that a new population of daughter cells with a greater growth advantage than their parental cells occurs, and that this cycle continues until a population of cells is present which displays none of the regulatory processes associated with normal cell growth and regulation. Slowly, the genetic mechanisms associated with changes in cellular control are being elucidated, and with it better avenues of intervention.

V. CONCLUSION

It has only been in the last 20 years that familial cancer has been widely recognized as an important genetic entity. During this period of time significant developments in our understanding of the changes that take place within a predisposed cell have occurred such that today, for many inherited cancer syndromes, the underlying cause can be precisely determined. In association with such advances predictive testing can now be performed on at-risk persons such that they no longer live with the uncertainty of not knowing if they have the predisposition. Persons who do have an increased risk of disease development can be accurately counseled and screened for the early detection of disease.

REFERENCES

1. **Easton, D. and Peto, J.** The contribution of inherited predisposition to cancer incidence. *Cancer Surveys* 9, 395, 1990.

2. **Price-Evans, D. A.** N-acetyltransferase. *Pharmacol. Ther.* 42, 157, 1989.
3. **Vineis, P.** Epidemiological models of carcinogenesis: the example of bladder cancer. Cancer Epidemiol. *Biomarkers Prev.* 1, 149, 1992.
4. **Mulvihill, J. J.** Clinical ecogenetics of human cancer. in *Familial Cancer*, Müller, Hj., Weber, W., and Kuttapa, T., Eds., S. Karger, Basel, 1985.
5. **Vineis, P.** The use of biomarkers in epidemiology: the example of bladder cancer. *Toxicol. Lett.* 463, 64, 1992.
6. **Knudson, A. G., Meadows, A. T., Nichols, W. W., and Hill, R.** Chromosomal deletion and retinoblastoma. *N. Engl. J. Med.* 295, 1120, 1976.
7. **Knudson, A. G.** Hereditary cancer, oncogenes, and antioncogenes. *Cancer Res.* 45, 1437, 1985.
8. **Würgler, F. E.** Recombination and gene conversion. *Mutat. Res.* 284, 3, 1992.
9. **Müller, Hj. and Scott, R. J.** Hereditary conditions in which a loss of heterozygosity may be important. *Mutat. Res.* 284, 15, 1992.
10. **Fearon, E. A. and Vogelstein, B.** A genetic model for colorectal tumorigenesis. *Cell* 61, 759, 1990.
11. **Fearon, E. R. and Jones, P. A.** Progressing toward a model for colorectal cancer development. *FASEB J.* 6, 2783, 1992.
12. **Bodmer, W. F., Bailey, C. J., Bodmer, J., Bussey, H. J. R., Ellis, A., Gormon, P., Lucibello, F. C., Murday, V. A., Rider, S. H., Scambler, P., Sheer, D., Solomon, E., and Spurr, N. K.** Localization of the gene for familial adenomatous polyposis on chromosome 5. *Nature* 328, 614, 1987.
13. **Nagase, H. and Nakamura, Y.** Mutations of the APC (adenomatous polyposis coli) gene. *Hum. Mutat.* 2, 425, 1993.
14. **Eng, C. and Ponder, B. A. J.** The role of gene mutations in the genesis of familial cancers. *FASEB J.* 7, 910, 1993.
15. **Harris, C. C. and Hollstein, M.** Clinical implications of the p53 tumor suppressor gene. *N. Engl. J. Med.* 329, 1318, 1993.
16. **Li, F. P. and Fraumeni, J. F., Jr.** Soft tissue sarcomas, breast cancer and other neoplasms: A familial syndrome? *Ann. Intern. Med.* 71, 747, 1969.
17. **Scott, R. J., Krummenacher, F., Mary, J.-L., Weber, W., Spycher, M., and Müller, Hj.** Vererbbare p53-Mutation bei einem Patienten mit Mehrfactumoren: Bedeutung für die genetische Beratung. *Schweiz. Med. Z.* 123, 1287, 1993.
18. **Malkin, D., Li, F. P., Strong, L. C., Fraumeni, J. F., Jr., Nelson, C. E., Kim, D. H., Kassel, J., Gryka, M. A., Bischoff, F. Z., Tainsky, M. A., and Friend, S. H.** Germ line p53 mutations in a familial syndrome of breast cancer, sarcomas, and other neoplasms. *Science* 250, 1233, 1990.
19. **Srivastava, S., Zou, Z., Pirollo, K., Blattner, W., and Chang, E. H.** Germ-line transmission of a mutated p53 gene in a cancer-prone family with Li-Fraumeni syndrome. *Nature* 348, 747, 1990.
20. **Li, F. P., Fraumeni, J. F., Jr., Mulvihill, J. J., Blattner, W. A., Dreyfus, M. G., Tucker, M. A., and Miller, R. W.** A cancer family syndrome in twenty four kindreds. *Cancer Res.* 48, 5358, 1988.
21. **Williams, W. R. and Strong, L. C.** Genetic epidemiology of soft tissue sarcomas in children, in *Familial Cancer*, Müller, Hj., Weber, W., and Kuttapa, T., Eds., S. Karger, Basel, 1985.
22. **Seto, E., Usheva, A., Zambetti, G. P., et al.** (1992) Wild-type p53 binds to the TATA-binding protein and represses transcription. *Proc. Natl. Acad. Sci. U.S.A.* 89, 12028, 1992.
23. **Vogelstein, B. and Kinzler, K. W.** p53 Function and dysfunction. *Cell* 70, 523, 1992.
24. **Aaltonen, L. A., Peltomäki, P., Leach, F. S., Sistonen, P., Rylkkanen, L., Mecklin, J. P., Järvinen, H., Powell, S. M., Jen, J., Hamilton, S. R., Petersen, G. M., Kinzler, K. W., Vogelstein, B., and de la Chapelle, A.** Clues to the pathogenesis of familial colorectal cancer. *Science* 260, 812, 1993.

25. **Peltomäki, P., Aaltonen, L. A., Sistonen, P., Pylkkanen, L., Mecklin, J. P., Jarvinen, H., Green, J. S., Jass, J. R., Weber, J. L., Leach, F. S., Petersen, G. M., Hamilton, S. R., de la Chappelle, A., and Vogelstein, B.** Genetic mapping of a locus predisposing to human colorectal cancer. *Science* 260, 810, 1993.

26. **Lindblom, A., Tannergärd, P., Werelius, B., and Nordenskjold, M.** Genetic mapping of a second locus predisposing to hereditary non-polyposis colon cancer. *Nat. Genet.* 5, 279, 1993.

27. **Thibodeau, S. N., Bren, G., and Schaid, D.** Microsatellite instability in cancer of the proximal colon. *Science* 269, 816, 1993.

28. **Fischel, R., Lescoe, M. K., Rao, M. R. S., Copeland, N. G., Jenkins, N. A., Garber, J., Kane, M., and Kolodner, R.** The human mutator gene homolog MSH2 and its association with hereditary nonpolyposis colon cancer. *Cell* 75, 1027, 1993.

29. **Leach, F. S., Nicolaides, N. C., Papadopoulos, N., Liu, B., Jen, J., et al.** Mutations of a mutS homolog in hereditary nonpolyposis colorectal cancer. *Cell* 75, 1215, 1993.

30. **Bronner, C. E., Baker, S. M., Morrison, P. T., Warren, G., Smith, L. G., Lescoe, M. K., Kane, M., Earabine, C., Lipford, J., Lindblom, A., Tannergard, P., Bollag, R. J., Godwin, A. R., Ward, D. C., Nordenskjold, M., Fishel, R., Kolodner, R., and Liskay, R. M.** Mutation in the DNA mismatch repair gene homologue hMLH1 is associated with hereditary non-polyposis colon cancer. *Nature* 368, 258, 1994.

31. **Papadopoulos, N., Nicolaides, N. C., Wei, Y.-F., Ruben, S. M., Carter, K. C., Rosen, C. A., Haseltine, W. A., Fleischmann, R. D., Fraser, C. M., Adams, M. D., Venter, J. C., Hamilton, S. R., Petersen, G. M., Watson, P., Lynch, H. T., Peltomäki, P., Mecklin, J.-P., de la Chapelle, A., Kinzler, K. W., and Vogelstein, B.** Mutation of a mutL homolog in hereditary colon cancer. *Science* 263, 1625, 1994.

32. **Nicolaides, N. C., Papadopoulos, N., Liu, B., Wei, Y.-F., Carter, K. C., Ruben, S. M., Rosen, C. A., Haseltine, W. A., Fleischmann, R. D., Fraser, C. M., Adams, M. D., Venter, J. C., Dunlop, M. G., Hamilton, S. R., Petersen, G. M., de la Chapelle, A., Vogelstein, B., and Kinzler, K. W.** Mutations of two PMS homologues in hereditary nonpolyposis colon cancer. *Nature* 371, 75, 1994.

33. **Parsons, R., Li, G.-U., Longley, M. J., Fang, W.-H., Papadopoulos, N., Jen, J., Chappelle, A., Kinzler, K. W., Vogelstein, B., and Modrich, P.** Hypermutability and mismatch repair deficiency in RER⁺ tumor cells. *Cell* 75, 1227, 1993.

34. **Kastan, M. B., Zhan, Q., El-Deiry, W. S., Carrier, F., Jacks, T., Walsh, W. V., Plunkett, B. S., Vogelstein, B., and Fornace, A. J., Jr.** A mammalian cell cycle checkpoint pathway utilizing p53 and GADD45 is defective in ataxia telangiectasia. *Cell* 71, 587, 1992.

35. **Latif, F., Tory, K., Gnarra, J., Yai, M., Duh, F.-M., Orcutt, M. L., Stackhouse, T., Kuzmin, I., Modi, W., Geil, L., Schmidt, L., Zhou, F., Li, H., Wei, M. H., Chen, F., Glenn, G., Choyke, P., Walther, M. M., Weng, Y., Duan, D.-S. R., Dean, M., Glavac, D., Richards, F. M., Crossey, P. A., Ferguson-Smith, M. A., Le Paslier, D., Chumakov, I., Cohen, D., Chinault, A. C., Maher, E. R., Linehan, W. M., Zbar, B., and Lerman, M. I.** Identification of the von Hippel-Lindau disease tumor suppressor gene. *Science* 260, 1317, 1993.

36. **Tory, K., Brauch, H., Linehan, M., Barba, D., Oldfield, E., Fillingkatz, M., Seizinger, B., Nakamura, Y., White, R., Marshal, F. F., Lerman, M. I., and Zbar, B.** Specific genetic change in tumors associated with von Hippel-Lindau disease. *J. Natl. Cancer Inst.* 81, 1097, 1989.

37. **Maher, E. A., Iselius, L., Yates, J. R. W., Littler, M., Benjamin, C., Harris, R., Sampson, J., Williams, A., Ferguson-Smith, M. A., and Morton, N.** Von Hippel disease: A genetic study. *J. Med. Genet.* 28, 443, 1991.

38. **Mulligan, L. M., Eng, C., Healey, C. S., Clayton, D., Kwok, J. B. J., Gardner, E., Ponder, M. A., Frilling, A., Jackson, C. E., Lehnert, H., Neumann, H. P. H., Thibodeau, S. N., and Pondes, B. A. J.** Specific mutations of the RET proto-oncogene are related to disease phenotype in MEN2A and FMTC. *Nat. Genet.* 6, 70, 1994.

39. **Gardner, E., Papi, L., Easton, D. F., Cummings, T., Jackson, C. E., Kaplan, M., Love, D. R., Mole, S. E., Moore, J. K., Mulligan, L. M., Norum, R. A., Ponder, M. A., Reichlin, S., Stall, G., Telenius, H., Telenius-Berg, M., Turnacliffe, A., and Ponder, B. A. J.** Genetic linkage studies map the multiple endocrine neoplasia type 2 loci to a small interval on chromosome 10q11.2. *Hum. Mol. Genet. 2*, 241, 1993.

40. **Radford, D. M., Ashley, S. W., Wells, S. A., Jr., and Gerhard, D. S.** Loss of heterozygosity of markers on chromosome 11 in tumors from patients with multiple endocrine neoplasia syndrome type 1. *Cancer Res. 50*, 6529, 1990.

41. **Brandi, M. L., Weber, G., Svennson, A., Falchetti, A., Tonelli, F., Castello, R., Furlani, L., Scappaticci, S., Fraccaro. M., and Larsson, C.** Homozygotes for the autosomal dominant neoplasia syndrome (MEN1). *Am. J. Hum. Genet. 53*, 1167, 1993.

42. **Bystrom, C., Larsson, C., Blomberg, C., Sandelin, K., Falkmer, U., Skogseid, B., Oberg, K., Werner, S., and Nordenskjold, M.** Localization of the MEN1 gene to a small region within chromosome 11 band q13 by deletion mapping in tumors. *Proc. Natl. Acad. Sci. U.S.A. 87*, 1968, 1990.

43. **Bale, A. E., Norton, J. A., Wong, E. L., Fryburg, J. S., Maton, P. N., Oldfield, E. H., Streeten, E., Aurbach, G. D., Brandi, M. L., Friedman, E., Spiegel, A. M., Taggart, R. T., and Marx, S. J.** Allelic loss on chromosome 11 in hereditary and sporadic tumors related to familial multiple endocrine neoplasia type I. *Cancer Res. 51*, 1154, 1991.

44. **Heutink, P., van der Mey, A. G. L., Sandkuijl, L. A., van Gils, A. P. G., Bardoel, A., Breedveld, G. J., van Vliet, M., Van Ommen, G. J., Cornelisse, C. J., Oastra, B. A., Weber, J. L., and Desilee, P.** A gene subject to genomic imprinting and responsible for hereditary paragangliomas maps to chromosome 11q23-qter. *Hum. Mol. Genet. 1*, 7, 1992.

45. **Mariman, E. C. M., van Beersum, S. E. C., Cremers, C. W. R. J., van Baars, F. M., and Ropers, H. H.** Analysis of a second family with hereditary non-chromaffin paragangliomas locates the underlying genes at the proximal region of chromosome 11q. *Hum. Genet. 91*, 357, 1993.

46. **Hall, J. M., Lee, M. K., Newman, B., Morrow, J. E., Anderson, L. A., Huey, B., and King, M.-C.** Linkage of early onset familial breast cancer to chromosome 17q21. *Science 250*, 1684, 1990.

47. **Easton, D. F., Bishop, D. T., Ford, D., Crockford, G. P., and the Breast Cancer Linkage Consortium.** Genetic linkage analysis in familial breast and ovarian cancer. Results from 214 families. *Am. J. Hum. Genet. 52*, 678, 1993.

48. **Bowcock, A. M., Anderson, L. A., Friedman, L. S., Black, D. M., Osborne-Lawrence, S., Rowell, S. E., Hall, J. M., Solomon, E., and King, M. C.** THRA1 and D17S183 flank an interval of <4cM for the breast-ovarian cancer gene. *Am. J. Hum. Genet. 52*, 718, 1993.

49. **Chamberlain, J. S., Boehnke, M., Frank, T. S., Kiousis, S., Xu, J., Guo, S.-W., Hauser, E. R., Norum, R. A., Helmbold, E. R., Markel, D. R., Keshavszi, S. M., Jackson, C. E., Calzone, K., Garber, J., Collins, F. S., and Weber, B. L.** BRCA1 maps proximal to D17S579 on chromosome 17q21 by genetic linkage analysis. *Am. J. Hum. Genet. 52*, 792, 1993.

50. **Cohen, B. B., Porter, D. E., Wallace, M. R., Carothers, A., and Steel, C. M.** Linkage of a major breast cancer gene on chromosome 17q12-21: results from 15 Edinburgh families. *Am. J. Hum. Genet. 52*, 723, 1993.

51. **Miki, Y., Swensen, J., Shattuck-Eldens, D., Futreal, P. A., Harshman, K., Tavtigian, S., Liu, Q., Cochran, C., Bennett, L. M., Ding, W., Bell, R., Rosenthal, J., Hussey, C., Tran, T., McClure, M., Frye, C., Hattier, T., Phelps, R., Haugen-Strano, A., Katcher, H., Yakumo, K., Gholami, Z., Shaffer, D., Stone, S., Bayer, S., Wray, C., Bogden, R., Dayananth, P., Ward, J., Tonin, P., Narod, S., Bristow, P. K., Norris, F. H., Helvering, N. L., Morrison, P., Rosteck, P., Lai, M., Berrett, J. C., Lewis, C., Neuhausen, S., Cannon-Albright, L., Goldgar, D., Wiseman, R., Kamb, A., and Skolnick, M. H.** A strong candidate for the breast ovarian cancer susceptibility gene BRCA1. *Science 266*, 66, 1994.

52. **Futreal, P. A., Liu, Q., Shattuck-Eidens, D., Cochran, C., Harshman, K., Tavtigian, S., Bennett, L.M., Haugen-Strano, A., Swensen, J., Miki, Y., Eddington, K., McClure, M., Frye, C., Weaver-Feldhaus, J., Ding, W., Gholami, Z., Soderkvist, P., Terry, L., Jhanwar, S., Berchuck, A., Iglehart, J. D., Marks, J., Ballinger, D. G., Barrett, J. C., Skolnick, M. H., Kamb, A., and Wiseman, R.** BRCA1 mutations in primary breast and ovarian carcinomas. *Science* 266, 120, 1994.

53. **Wooster, R., Neuhausen, S. L., Mangion, J., Quirk, Y., Ford, D., Collins, N., Nguyen, K., Seal, S., Tran, T., Averill, D., Fields, P., Marshall, G., Narod, S., Lenoir, G. M., Lynch, H., Feuteun, J., Devilee, P., Cornelisse, C. J., Menko, F., Daly, P. A., Ormiston, W., McManus, R., Pye, C., Lewis, C. M., Cannon-Albright, L. A., Peto, J., Ponder, B. A. J., Skolnick, M. H., Easton, D. F., Goldgar, D. E., and Stratton, M. R.** Localization of a breast cancer susceptibility gene, BRCA2, to chromosome 13q12-13. *Science* 265, 2088, 1994.

54. **Harris, H., Miller, O. J., Klein, G., Worst, P., and Tachibana, T.** Suppression of malignancy by cell fusion. *Nature* 223, 363, 1969.

55. **Chen, P.-L., Chen, Y., Bookstein, R., and Lee, W. H.** Genetic mechanisms of tumor suppression by the human p53 gene. *Science* 250, 1576, 1990.

56. **Yin, Y., Tainsky, M. A., Bischoff, F. Z., Strong, L. C., and Wahl, G. M.** Wild-type p53 restores cell cycle control and inhibits gene amplification in cells with mutant p53 alleles. *Cell* 70, 937, 1992.

57. **Shipman, R., Schraml, P., Colombi, M., Raefle, G., and Ludwig, C. U.** Loss of heterozygosity on chromosome 11p13 in primary bladder carcinoma. *Hum. Genet.* 91, 455, 1993.

58. **Fearon, E. A. and Vogelstein, B.** A genetic model for colorectal tumorigenesis. *Cell* 61, 759, 1990.

59. **Malkin, D., Jolly, K. W., Barbier, N., Look, A. T., Friend, S. H., Gebhardt, M. C., Andersen, T. I., Borrensen, A.-L., Li, F. P., Garber, J., and Strong, L. C.** Germline mutations of the p53 tumor suppressor gene in children and young adults with second malignant neoplasms. *Nature* 326, 1309, 1992.

60. **Cairns, J.** Mutation selection and the natural history of cancer. *Nature* 255, 197, 1975.

61. **Peto, R., Roe, F. J. C., Lee, P. N., Levy, L., and Clark, J.** Cancer and aging in mice and men. *Br. J. Cancer* 32, 411, 1975.

62. **Weinberg, R. A.** Oncogenes, anti-oncogenes, and molecular basis of multiple carcinogenesis. *Cancer Res.* 49, 3713, 1989.

63. **Knudson, A. G., Jr.** Mutation and cancer: statistical study of retinoblastoma. *Proc. Natl. Acad. Sci. U.S.A.* 68, 820, 1971.

64. **Collins, V. P. and James, C. D.** Gene and chromosomal alterations associated with the development of human glioblastomas. *FASEB J.* 7, 926, 1993.

65. **Bischoff, F. Z., Yim, S. O., Pathak, S., Grant, G., Sicilano, M. J., Giovanella, B. C., Strong, L. C., and Tainsky, M. A.** Spontaneous abnormalities in normal fibroblasts from patients with Li-Fraumeni cancer syndrome: aneuploidy and immortalization. *Cancer Res.* 50, 7979, 1990.

66. **Ruiz, J. C. and Wahl, G. M.** Chromosomal destabilization during gene amplification. *Mol. Cell. Biol.* 10, 3056, 1990.

67. **Livingstone, L. R., White, A., Sprouse, L., Livanos, E., Jacks, T., and Tlsty, T. D.** Altered cell cycle arrest and gene amplification potential accompany loss of wild type p53. *Cell* 70, 923, 1992.

68. **Hartwell, L.** Defects in checkpoint may be responsible for the genomic instability of cancer cells. *Cell* 71, 543, 1992.

69. **Yokota, J. and Sugimura, T.** Multiple steps in carcinogenesis involving alterations of multiple tumor suppressor genes. *FASEB J.* 7, 920, 1993.

Chapter 2

ENVIRONMENTAL FACTORS IN FAMILIAL CANCER

Walter Weber

TABLE OF CONTENTS

I. INTRODUCTION

If familial aggregation is observed, it is necessary to decide whether such aggregation is a result of environmental or genetic factors or both. Careful consideration has to be given to environmental factors that aggregate in families before implicating genetic mechanisms.[1] Agents such as infections, drugs, or radiation in prior generations can influence the occurrence of single gene disorders. Mendelian conditions may not manifest clinically unless accompanied by specific environmental exposures, e.g., malignant lymphoma induced by the Epstein-Barr Virus (EBV) in the X-linked lymphoproliferative syndrome.[2]

17

II. MECHANISMS

Increasing evidence suggests that cancer initiation and progression are a multistep process resulting from the accumulation of genetic events over time.[3] Understanding the molecular controls of the cellular response to DNA damaging agents would provide insights into carcinogenesis. Critical responses to carcinogens that could influence cellular transformation are likely to include: (1) the ability to metabolize a procarcinogen to a carcinogen (increased risk) or a carcinogen to an inactive metabolite (decreased risk); (2) the ability to repair damage to the DNA; (3) the effects on cell cycle progression and the timing of cell cycle arrests relative to damage repair; and (4) the factors that influence cell survival following DNA damage.[4] It may be that the subtle differences in response among individuals are important variables for determining who will get cancer. Experimental techniques allow the manipulation of the genetic make-up of an animal to investigate the physiologic ramifications of disruption of genes that are likely to be involved in DNA damage responses and to evaluate their potential roles in carcinogenesis. Mice can be generated in which one or both copies of a repair gene are disrupted by homologous recombination.[5] Loss of p53 function greatly increases cancer incidence in mice.[6] Heterozygous *p53* mice are more susceptible to tumor development after treatment with the carcinogen dimethylnitrosamine. They are extremely susceptible to radiation-induced tumorigenesis.[78] Homozygous *p53*-deficient mice develop malignancies so rapidly that the addition of the carcinogen did not alter their outcome; presumably this was due to the latency period required for development of the carcinogen-induced tumor. Thus *p53* acts as a tumor suppressor by preventing the propagation of DNA damage to daughter cells.[7]

As with most human illnesses, cancer suceptibility is likely to be the result of interactions between the environment and an individual's genotype/phenotype.[76,77] The importance of the genetic component will likely depend on the strength of the environmental influence.

The development of statistical tools for studying familial disease has until recently progressed along different lines for epidemiologists and geneticists.[8] While epidemiologists have concentrated on environmental and lifestyle risk factors and sometimes assessed these factors in conjunction with familial factors, geneticists have concentrated on the possible genetic mechanism without paying due attention to environmental risk factors. Because family members tend to share genes, environments, and lifestyles, focusing on one of these factors in the analysis of family data may lead to results confounded by one of the others. The recent statistical methods for analyzing family data are merging the approaches of the epidemiologists and geneticists.[79]

A new approach to establishing carcinogen exposure is pursued in molecular epidemiology. It explore possibilities to detect signal changes or "markers" in DNA, chromosomes, and other cellular targets years before cancer appears.[9,10]

It is to be expected that every carcinogen can lead to familial cancer clustering, such as familial mesothelioma[11] or familial urinary bladder cancer.[12] The IARC Monographs Program in Lyon, France aims to identify agents that increase the risk of cancer in exposed humans.[13] Working groups of invited experts in carcinogenesis follow guidelines established during several consultative meetings in formulating their evaluations.

III. GENERAL ASPECTS

Exposure to carcinogens and/or their inhibitors is the key determinant of cancer occurrence.[14] Genetic factors act in combination with such environmental factors. Good examples of the existence of environmental-genetic interactions are tumors in *repair-related inherited disorders* (Table 1). Ataxia telangiectasia (AT) is a rare autosomal recessive disorder in which individuals exhibit cerebellar ataxia, oculocutaneous telangiectasia, immunological defects, abnormal radiation sensitivity, and predisposition to cancer, particularly breast cancer.[15] There are at least five clinically indistinguishable complement groups. Group A has been located in the long arm of chromosome 11 and the gene ATM isolated.[16]

Bloom syndrome (BS) is a rare, autosomal recessive disorder exhibiting numerous clinical features including sensitivity to sunlight, growth retardation, immunological disorders, and a predisposition to cancer at a relatively young age. DNA ligase I activity is clearly reduced in BS cells, but the underlying defect is not yet known.[17] Fanconi anemia (FA) is an autosomal recessive disorder characterized by progressive pancytopenia, a diverse assortment of congenital malformations, and a predisposition to the development of malignancies, particularly acute myeloid leukemia. There is evidence for at least four FA genes.[18] Xeroderma pigmentosum (XP), a rare autosomal recessive hereditary disease, results from a defect in nucleotide excision repair of ultraviolet-damaged DNA. XP patients are extremely sensitive to sunlight and suffer from a high incidence of skin cancers.[19] Cell fusion studies have identified seven XP complementation groups, A - G. Group D is of particular interest as mutations in this gene can also cause Cockayne's syndrome and trichothiodystrophy.[20,21]

TABLE 1
CANCER-PRONE
REPAIR-RELATED
INHERITED DISORDERS

Ataxia telangiectasia	(AT)
Bloom syndrome	(BS)
Cockayne syndrome	(CS)
Fanconi anemia	(FA)
Xeroderma pigmentosum	(XP)

A. SKIN CANCER

There is considerable interest and a generalized lack of data from population-based studies concerning the incidence of skin neoplasms, particularly
non-melanocytic skin cancers. This is because of the well-known difficulties
in obtaining accurate information on these often trivial tumors, and the problem
of defining "incident" cancers when a single individual develops many tumors.
The large majority of basal and squamous cell cancers arising on the head and
neck confirms the importance of long-term ultraviolet light exposure; the
relative excess of squamous cell as compared to basal cell neoplasms on the
upper limb may suggest the role of exposure to other carcinogens; and the
proportional excess of melanomas on the trunk in males and lower limb in
females further indicates that intermittent exposure to sunlight is probably the
relevant etiologic factor for melanocytic skin neoplasms.[22]

Environmental as well as host characteristics play a role in the development
of skin cancer.[23] Skin type, sunburn sensitivity, the presence of numerous and/or
clinically atypical nevi, and ultraviolet light exposure are major risk factors for
cutaneous melanoma. A positive family history for melanoma increases the
relative risk of manifesting the disease by 2–8 times the average incidence.[24]
Approximately 8–12 % of all melanomas occur within families in which two
or more members have this malignancy. Complex multistep modeling of the
data available may be helpful in characterizing the genetic patterns of cutaneous melanoma.[25] Nevoid basal cell carcinoma syndrome (Gorlin syndrome) is
an autosomal dominant disorder, characterized primarily by multiple basal cell
carcinomas, epithelium-lined jaw cysts, and palmar and plantar pits. Loss of
heterozygosity studies and linkage analysis have mapped the gene to chromosome 9q and suggest that it is a tumor suppressor.[80]

B. GEOGRAPHICAL VARIATIONS

Geographical patterns of cancer distribution are similar in males and females, strongly suggesting that factors affecting such geographical differences
operate in similar fashion in both sexes.[14] Similarities are observed in certain
pairs of cancers of sex-specific sites (e.g., cancer of the testis and ovary, and
cancer of the penis and cervix) suggesting that risk factors including genetic
predisposition may be commonly operating.[14]

Observing cancer patterns in migrants may clarify etiologic issues. Migration of a population from one environment to another provides an example of
a "natural experiment", allowing the risk of disease to be compared in populations of similar genetic background living in different environments.[26] Dis-
similarities in the pattern of cancer occurrence in different countries are im-
pressive.[13] Groups of neighboring countries tend to show rather similar patterns
(e.g., oral cancer in India and Sri Lanka, cervical cancer in most of Latin
America, stomach cancer in China, Japan, and Korea, liver cancer in most
countries in Africa and Asia, malignant lymphoma in the Middle East, gallbladder cancer in Bolivia and New Mexico). Environmental conditions as well

as genetic factors must be considered in interpreting such phenomena. Such regional cancer patterns suggest the desirability of a regional aproach in global cancer control programs.[14]

IV. FAMILIAL AGGREGATION OF FREQUENT MALIGNANCIES

A. FAMILIAL LUNG CANCER

Lung cancer is the most common cancer, accounting for 11.8% of all cancers in the world.[27] Lung cancer is the single most important tobacco-related disease not appreciably influenced by alcohol or other major lifestyle risk factors, and is a major cause of illness and premature death as well as of health-related costs.[28] Lung cancer mortality is close to incidence because of poor survival rates, and the seriousness of the disease makes the diagnosis more reliable than for other conditions. Active cigarette smoking is the principal cause of lung cancer.[29] But passive smoking also is causally associated with lung cancer in adults.[30]

As far back as 1963, Tokuhata and Lilienfeld[31] presented data showing the familial aggregation of lung cancer, suggesting the possible interactions of genes, shared environment, and common life-style factors in the etiology of lung cancer. They compared lung cancer deaths in controls who were matched for age, sex, race, and neighborhood. In their study, cases' relatives were two to three times as likely as controls' relatives to die of lung cancer after adjusting for the smoking habits of the relatives.

Lynch et al.[32] studied detailed cancer family histories on 254 consecutively ascertained probands with histologically verified lung cancer and 231 probands with other smoking-related cancers who were under medical evaluation at the Creighton Oncology Clinic. Results disclosed a lack of statistical evidence for an increased risk in lung cancer per se when only lung cancer in relatives was considered. However, a significant increase was observed in cancers of all anatomic sites among the relatives of lung cancer probands.

Horwitz et al.[33] conducted a case-control study with 112 women affected by lung cancer and 224 controls. Patients who never smoked but had a positive family history had an odds ratio of 5.7; patients who smoked but had a negative family history had an odds ratio of 15.1; and patients who smoked and had a positive family history had an odds ratio of almost 30.

Data pointing to a synergistic action of factors are also reported from Japan.[34] In a case-control analysis, the relative risk of lung cancer was 1.7 for those subjects with a family history alone, 2.2 for those with a smoking habit alone, and 3.6 for those with both a family history and who smoked.

A population-based case-control study of 336 female patients with adenocarcinoma of the lung and an equal number of neighborhood controls revealed a significant fourfold excess risk associated with a family history of lung cancer.[35] No excess risk was observed for family histories of other cancers. Sellers et al.[36] reported an interesting gene-environment interaction using segregation analyses on 337 families, each ascertained through a lung cancer proband. In patients at age of 50, 27% of the lung cancers are attributable to a Mendelian gene alone, 42% to the joint effect of a gene and smoking, 27% to smoking alone, and 4% to neither the alleged gene nor smoking. In patients at age 70, however, only 9% of the lung cancers can be attributed to an alleged gene, 13% to the joint effect of the gene and smoking, 72% to smoking alone, and 6% to neither the alleged gene nor smoking.

Caporaso et al.[37] reported evidence that the ability to metabolize debrisoquine is a major determinant of susceptibility to lung cancer. Individuals who were extensive metabolizers of debrisoquine were at significantly greater risk of lung cancer than those who were poor or intermediate metabolizers (odds ratio = 6.1; 90% confidence interval = 2.2–17.1).

Familial lung cancer occurs in association with limb and dental abnormalities and a balanced chromosome 13 to 14 translocation.[38] It is also a possible element of the Li-Fraumeni syndrome.[39]

1. Treatment

Non-small-cell lung cancer (NSCLC) accounts for 75% of lung cancer cases. Most patients present with advanced, unresectable disease for which radiation therapy and/or chemotherapy is the standard form of treatment. Only 25% of the patients present with resectable disease. They have a 5-year survival of 50%. In the other patients it is less than 10%. New drugs are needed.[40]

Small-cell lung cancer (SCLC) accounts for 25% of lung cancer cases and tends to progress very quickly. Even in patients who receive systematic chemotherapy, with or without radiation, the median survival is only 11 months.[41] It is important to pursue treatment strategies that focus on the palliative effect of therapy, including quality of life studies.

2. Prevention

Smoking is the leading cause of preventable, premature death. Not starting to smoke and smoking cessation are clearly beneficial in reducing the risk of dying from smoking-related diseases. Nicotine replacement therapies are effective components of strategies to help people stop smoking.[42] Heredity has a moderate influence on smoking behavior.[43] A family history of smoking increases the risk that a child will become a smoker. Such children should be targets for intensive preventive efforts. Dietary beta carotene, raw fruit and vegetables, and vitamin E supplements reduce the risk of lung cancer in smoking and nonsmoking men and women.[44]

B. FAMILIAL LIVER CANCER

Hepatocellular carcinoma (HCC) is frequent in sub-Saharan Africa, eastern and southeastern Asia, Melanesia, and southern Europe.[27] Chronic hepatitis B virus (HBV) has been shown to be an etiologic factor.[45] Chronic infection with

HBV and hepatitis C virus (HCV) are carcinogenic to humans.[46] High levels of aflatoxin in the diet may also play a role.[47] HCC is associated with hepatitis, cirrhosis, and parasitic infections.[48] Interactions between chronic HBV infection and p53 mutations are suggested.[49] A putative tumor suppressor gene for HCC without cirrhosis may be located on chromosome 5q.[50]

1. Family Reports

Kaplan and Cole[51] as well as Hagstrom and Baker[52] reported HCC in three male siblings. Ohbayashi et al.[53] reported three kindreds with six HCC. Denison et al.[54] described two brothers and Tepfer[55] a third brother with HCC who gave the history that their father had died of cancer of the liver at the age of 60. Velasco et al.[56] described a family from Chile involving two brothers with HCC. Clustering of HBV infection is commonly present in family members of patients with HCC.[57] Lynch et al.[58] presented a family in Thailand in which histologically verified HCC was found in a mother and two of her four sons, all of whom were concordant for HBV infection.

2. Large Series

Of 1065 families with HCC in China, 41% had two or more affected relatives.[59] If either parent suffered from HCC, their children will be affected in 35%.[59] Clustering of HCC is reported in Alaskan native families, in a population where HBV infection is common.[60]

3. Treatment

Few patients fulfill criteria for a curative surgical attempt such as a solitary lesion limited to one lobe of the liver and absence of cirrhosis, jaundice, or ascites.[61] Palliative measures include radiation, systemic and regional chemotherapy, analgesia, and care.[61]

4. Prevention

Proper control of intrafamilial spread of HBV infection may aid in decreasing the incidence of chronic liver disease and of primary HCC. One promising approach is HBV vaccination. Large-scale vaccination projects have been initiated in high incidence areas such as Qidong County of China[62] and The Gambia in Africa.[63]

5. Hepatoblastoma

Hepatoblastoma is the most frequent primary malignant tumor of the liver in children. Hereditary conditions such as neurofibromatosis may predispose individuals to it.[64] Childhood hepatoblastoma may also be an associated feature of familial adenomatous polyposis.[65] Familial clustering of hepatoblastoma is reported.[66] Malformations such as Beckwith-Wiedemann syndrome can be associated with hepatoblastoma.[67] Early diagnosis and aggressive surgery (including liver transplantation) are advocated for the treatment of hepatoblastoma.

C. FAMILIAL CERVIX CANCER

Cervix cancer is the most frequent cancer of women in almost all of the developing areas.[27] There is strong epidemiological evidence that certain types of human papillomavirus (HPV) cause cervical cancer,[68] and HPV DNA has been found in up to 90% of women with cervical cancer.[69]

It is surprising that few studies have addressed the familial aggregation of cervix cancer. In a 1966 study, Rotkin found that male relatives of cervical cancer patients had an excess of skin cancer.[70] A high risk of a family history of cervix cancer was observed in adenosquamous cervix cancer (RR = 9.9), though based on only two cases, while the corresponding risks for squamous cell cancer and adenocarcinoma were 3.1 and 2.5, respectively.[71] Women with HLA-DQw3 are at high risk of squamous cell cervix cancer.[72] Defense by the immune system against tumors induced by viruses is known to be important in experimental animals.[72] Specific HLA class II haplotypes may influence the immune response to specific HPV-encoded epitopes and affect the risk of cervical neoplasia.[73]

1. Treatment

Surgery and radiation therapy have a similar curative and palliative potential, either alone or in combination.[74] The optimal situation is to be treated in institutions that have personnel and equipment suitable for either type of therapy and for selection of therapy to be a joint decision of the surgeon, the radiation oncologist, and the patient. Chemotherapy has a limited and only palliative role.

2. Prevention

Of all the female genital cancers, only cervical cancer can be reliably prevented by an effective, inexpensive screening technique that allows detection and treatment of precancerous conditions. Many deaths due to cervical cancer could be prevented if women would avail themselves of routine screening with cervical cytologic analysis. Screening should start at about the age of 20 with a screening interval of 2 to 5 years.[75]

REFERENCES

1. **Lilienfeld, A. M.,** Formal discussion of genetic factors in the etiology of cancer: an epidemiologic view, *Cancer Res.* 25, 1330–1335, 1965.
2. **Hayoz, D., Lenoir, G. M., Nicole, A., Pugin, P., and Regamey, C.,** X-linked lymphoproliferative syndrome. Identification of a large family in Switzerland, *Am. J. Med.* 84, 529–534, 1988.
3. **Schwechheimer, K. and Cavenee, W. K.,** Genetics of cancer predisposition and progression. *Clin. Invest.* 71, 488–502, 1993.

4. **Kastan, M. B.,** Experimental models of human carcinogenesis, *Nat. Genet.* 5, 207–208, 1993.
5. **McWhir, J., Selfridge, J., Harrison, D. J., Squires, S., and Melton, D. W.,** Mice with DNA repair gene (ERCC-1) deficiency have elevated levels of p53, liver nuclear abnormalities and die before weaning. *Nat. Genet.* 5, 217–223, 1993.
6. **Harvey, M., McArthur, M. J., Montgomery, C. A., Jr., Butel, J. S., Bradley, A., and Donehower, L. A.,** Spontaneous and carcinogen-induced tumorigenesis in p53-deficient mice. *Nat. Genet.* 5, 225–229, 1993.
7. **Purdie, C. A., Harrison, D. J., Peter, A., Dobbie, L., White, S., Howie, S. E. M., Salter, D. M., Bird, C. C., Wyllie, A. M., Hooper, M. L., and Clarke, A. R.,** Tumour incidence, spectrum and ploidy in mice with a large deletion in the p53 gene. *Oncogene* 9, 603–609, 1994.
8. **Bonney, G. E.,** Interactions of genes, environment, and life-style in lung cancer development. *J. Natl. Cancer Inst.* 82, 122–123, 1990.
9. **Perera, F. P.,** Molecular epidemiology: A new tool in assessing risks of environmental carcinogens. *CA-A Ca. J. Clin.* 40, 277–288, 1990.
10. **Correa, P.,** The new era of cancer epidemiology. *Cancer Epidemiol. Biomarkers Prev.* 1, 5–11, 1991.
11. **Hammar, S. P., Bockus, D., Remington, F., Freidman, S., and Lazerte, G.** Familial mesothelioma: A report of two families. *Hum. Pathol.* 20, 107–112, 1989.
12. **Purtilo, D. T., McCarthy, B., Yang, J. P. S., Friedell, G. H., and the Worcester Urology Group,** Familial urinary bladder cancer. *Semin. Oncol.* 6, 254–256, 1979.
13. **IARC Biennial Report 1992–1993.** *International Agency for Research on Cancer*, 1993. Lyon, France.
14. **Hirayama, T.,** Genetic epidemiology of cancer, in *Genetic Epidemiology*, Lynch H. T. and Hirayama T., Eds., CRC Press, Boca Raton, FL, 1989, 69–101.
15. **Swift, M., Morrell, D., Massey, R. B., and Chase, C. L.,** Incidence of cancer in 161 families affected by ataxia-telangiectasia. *N. Engl. J. Med.* 325, 1831–1836, 1991.
16. **Gatti, R. A.,** Localizing the genes for ataxia-telangiectasia: a human model for inherited cancer susceptibility. *Adv. Cancer Res.*, 56, 77–104, 1991.
17. **Llerena, J. C. and Murer-Orlando, M.,** Bloom syndrome and ataxia telangiectasia. *Semin. Hematol.* 28, 95–103, 1991.
18. **Strathdee, C. A., Duncan, A. M. V., and Buchwald, M.,** Evidence for a least four Fanconi anaemia genes including FACC on chromosome 9. *Nat. Genet.* 1, 196–198, 1992.
19. **Kraemer, K. H., Lee, M. M., and Scotto, J.,** Xeroderma pigmentosum cutaneous, ocular and neurologic abnormalities in 830 published cases. *Arch. Dermatol.* 123, 241–250, 1987.
20. **Wood, R. D.,** Seven genes for three diseases. *Nature* 350, 190, 1991.
21. **Sung, P., Baily, V., Weber, C., Thompson, L. H., Prakash, L., and Prakash, S.,** Human xeroderma pigmentosum group D gene encodes a DNA helicase. *Nature* 365, 852–855, 1993.
22. **Levi, F., La Vecchia, C., Te, V. C., and Mezzanotte, G.,** Descriptive epidemiology of skin cancer in the Swiss canton of Vaud. *Int. J. Cancer* 42, 811–816, 1988.
23. **Fusaro, R. M.,** The environment and cancer-associated genodermatoses, in *Genetic Epidemiology of Cancer*, Lynch, H. T. and Hirayama T., Eds., CRC Press, Boca Raton, FL, 1989, chap. 11.
24. **Duggleby, W. F., Stoll, H., Priore, R. L., Greenwald, P., and Graham, S. A.,** A genetic analysis of melanoma: polygenetic inheritance as a threshold trait, *Am. J. Epidemiol.* 114, 1363–1372, 1981.
25. **Duke, D., Castresana, J., Lucchina, L., Lee, T. II., Sober, A. J., Carey, W. P., Elder, D. E., and Barnhill, R. L.,** Familial cutaneous melanoma and two-mutational-event modeling, *Cancer* 72, 3239–3243, 1993.
26. **Parkin, D. M.,** Studies of cancer in migrant populations: mehtods and interpretation. *Rev. Epidemiol. Santé Publ.* 40, 410–424, 1992.

27. **Parking, D. M., Pisani, P., and Ferlay, J.,** Estimates of the worldwide incidence of eighteen major cancers in 1985. *Int. J. Cancer* 54, 594–606, 1993.

28. **Boffetta, P., La Vecchia, C., Levi, F., and Lucchini, F.,** Mortality patterns and trends for lung cancer and other tobacco-related cancers in the Americas, 1955–1989. *Int. J. Epidemiol.* 22, 377–384, 1993.

29. **U.S. Department of Health and Human Services.** The health benefits of smoking cessation. A report of the surgeon general. DHHS Publ. No. (CDC) 90–8416, 1990.

30. **Environmental Protection Agency.** Respiratory health effects of passive smoking: Lung cancer and other disorders. Washington, D.C., Office of Health and Environmental Assessment, 1–4, 1992.

31. **Tokuhata, G. K. and Lilienfeld, A. M.,** Familial aggregation of lung cancer in humans, *J. Natl. Cancer Inst.* 30, 289–312, 1963.

32. **Lynch H. T., Kimberling, W. J., Markivicka, S. E., Biscone, K. A., Lynch, J. F., Whorton, E., and Mailliard, J.,** Genetics and smoking-associated cancers. *Cancer* 57, 1640–1646, 1986.

33. **Horwitz, R. I., Smaldone, L. F., and Viscoli, C. M.,** An ecogenetic hypothesis for lung cancer in women. *Arch. Intern. Med.* 148, 2609–2612, 1988.

34. **Ogawa, J., Tominaga, S., and Kato, I.,** Family clustering of cancer: analysis of cancer registry data. *Gann. Monogr. Cancer Res.* 35, 135–144, 1988.

35. **Wu, A. H., Yu, M. C., Thomas, D. C., Pike, M. C., and Henderson, B. E.,** Personal and family history of lung disease as risk factors for adenocarcinoma of the lung. *Cancer Res.* 48, 7279–7284, 1988.

36. **Sellers, T. A., Bailey-Wilson, J. E., Elston, R. C., Wilson, A. F., Elston, G. Z., Ooi, W. L., and Rothschild, H.,** Evidence for Mendelian inheritance in the pathogenesis of lung cancer. *J. Natl. Cancer Inst.* 82, 1272–1279, 1990.

37. **Caporaso, N. E., Tucker, M. A., Hoover, R. N., Hayes, R. B., Pickle, L. W., Issaq, H. J., Muschik, G. M., Gren-Gallo, L., Buivys, D., Aisner, S., Resan, J. H., Trump, B. F., Tollerud, D., Weston, A., and Harris C. C.,** Lung cancer and the drbrisoquine metabolic phenotype. *J. Natl. Cancer Inst.* 82, 1264–1272, 1990.

38. **Goffman, T. E., Hassinger, D. D., and Mulvihill, J. J.,** Familial respiratory tract cancer. *JAMA* 247, 1020–1023, 1982.

39. **Malkin, D., Li, F. P., Strong, L. C., Fraumeni, J. F. Jr., Nelson, C. E., Kim, D. H., Kassel, J., Gryka, M. A., Bischoff, F. Z., Tainsky, M. A., and Friend S. H.,** Germ-line p53 mutations in a familial syndrome of breast cancer, sarcomas, and other neoplasms. *Science* 250, 1233–1238, 1990.

40. **Feigal, E. G., Christian, M., Cheson, B., Grever, M., and Friedmann, A.,** New chemotherapeutic agents in non-small-cell lung cancer. *Semin. Oncol.* 20, 185–201, 1993.

41. **Hansen, H. H.,** Management of small-cell cancer of the lung. *Lancet* 339, 846–849, 1992.

42. **Silagy, C., Mant, D., Fowler, G., and Lodge, M.,** Meta-analysis of efficacy of nicotine replacement therapies in smoking cessation. *Lancet* 343, 139–142, 1994.

43. **Carmelli, D., Swan, G. E., Robinette, D., and Fabsitz, R.,** Genetic influence on smoking — a study of male twins. *N. Engl. J. Med.* 327, 829–833, 1992.

44. **Mayne, S. T., Janerich, D. T., Greenwald, P., Chorost, S., Tucci, C., Zaman, M. B., Melamed, M. R., Kiely, M., and McKneally, M. F.,** Dietary beta carotene and lung cancer risk in U.S. nonsmokers. *J. Natl. Cancer Inst.* 86, 33–38, 1994.

45. **Beasley, R. P.,** Hepatitis B virus. The major etiology of hepatocellular carcinoma. *Cancer* 61, 1942–1956, 1988.

46. **IARC Monographs,** Volume 59, WHO, Geneva, 1993.

47. **Wogan, G. N.,** Aflatoxins as risk factors for hepatocellular carcinoma in humans. *Cancer Res.*, 52, 2114s–2118s, 1992.

48. **Oberfield, R. A., Steele, G., Jr., Gollan, J., and Sherman, D.,** Liver cancer. *CA. Cancer J. Clin.* 39, 206–218, 1989.

49. **Hsia, C. C., Kleiner, D. E., Axiotis, C. A., DiBiscegli, A., Nomura, A. M. Y., Stemmermann, G. N., and Tabor, E.,** Mutations of p53 gene in hepatocellular carcinoma: roles of hepatitis B virus and aflatoxin contamination in the diet. *J. Natl. Cancer Inst.* 84, 1638–1641, 1992.

50. **Ding, S. F., Delhanty, J. D. A., Dooley, J. S., Bowles, L., Wood, C. B., and Habib, N. A.,** The putative tumor suppressor gene on chromosome 5q for hepatocellular carcinoma is distinct from the MCC and APC genes. *Cancer Detection Prev.* 17, 405–409, 1993.

51. **Kaplan, L. and Cole, S. L.,** Fraternal primary hepatocellular carcinoma in three male, adult siblings. *Am. J. Med.* 39, 305–311, 1965.

52. **Hagstrom, R. and Baker, T. D.,** Primary hepatocellular carcinoma in three male siblings. *Cancer* 22, 142–150, 1968.

53. **Ohbayashi, A., Okochi, K., and Mayumi, M.,** Familial clustering of asymptomatic carriers of Australia antigen and patients with chronic liver disease or primary liver cancer. *Gastroenterology* 62, 618–625, 1972.

54. **Denison, E. K., Peters, R. L., and Reynolds, T. B.,** Familial hepatoma with hepatitis-associated antigen. *Ann. Intern. Med.* 74, 391–394, 1971.

55. **Tepfer, B. D.,** Hepatoma and HAA. Letter. *Ann. Intern. Med.* 76, 145–146, 1972.

56. **Velasco, M., Sorensen, R., Daiber, A., Carmona, A., and Kotz, R.,** Primary carcinoma of the liver associated with Australia antigen. Letter. *Lancet* 1, 1183–1184, 1971.

57. **Tong, M. J., Weiner, J. M., Ashcaval, M. W., and Vyas, G. N.,** Evidence for clustering of hepatitis B virus infection in families of patients with primary hepatocellular carcinoma. *Cancer* 44, 2338–2342, 1979.

58. **Lynch, H. T., Srivatanskul, P., Phornthutkul, K., and Lynch, J. F.,** Familial hepatocellular carcinoma in an endemic area of Thailand. *Cancer Genet. Cytogenet.* 11, 11–18, 1984.

59. **Qi, X. D.,** Personal communication. Third UICC strategy meeting on familial cancer in Asia and Oceania, Kobe, Japan, 1993.

60. **Alberts, S. R., Lanier, A. P., McMahon, B. J., Harpster, A., Bulkow, L. R., Heyward, W. L., and Murray, C.,** Clustering of hepatocellular carcinoma in Alaska native families. *Genet. Epidemiol.* 8, 127–139, 1991.

61. **Oberfield, R. A., Steele, G., Gollan, J. L., and Sherman, D.,** Liver cancer. *CA-A Cancer J. Clinic.* 39, 206–218, 1989.

62. **Sun, Z. (T.), Zhu, Y., Stjernsward, J., Hilleman, M., Collins, R., Zhew, Y., Hsia, C. C., Lu, J., Huang, F., Ni, Z., Ni, T., Liu, G. T., Yu, Z., Liu, Y., Chen, J. M., and Peto, R.,** Design and compliance of HBV vaccination trial on newborns to prevent hepatocellular carcinoma and 5-year results of its pilot study. *Cancer Detection Prev.* 15, 313–318, 1991.

63. **The Gambia Hepatitis Study Group,** The Gambia hepatitis intervention study. *Cancer Res.* 47, 5781–5787, 1987.

64. **Fraumeni, J. F., Miller, R. W., and Hill, J. A.,** Primary carcinoma of the liver in childhood: an epidemiologic study. *J. Natl. Cancer Inst.* 40, 1087–1099, 1968.

65. **Li, F. P., Thurber, W. A., Seddon, J., and Holmes, G. E.,** Hepatoblastoma in families with polyposis coli. *JAMA* 257, 2475–2477, 1987.

66. **Riikonen, P., Tuominen, L., Seppä, A., and Perkkiö, M.,** Simultaneous hepatoblastoma in identical male twins. *Cancer* 66, 2429–2431, 1990.

67. **Haas, O. A., Zoubek, A., Grümayer, E. R., Ferstl, G., and Gardner, H.,** The Wiedemann-Beckwith syndrome. Clinical characteristics, constitutional chromosome anomalies and tumor incidence. *Klin. Pädiatr.* 199, 283–291, 1987.

68. **Jha, P. K. S., Beral, V., Peto, J., Hack, S., Hermon, C., Deacon, J., Mant, D., Chilvers, C., Vessey, M. P., Pike, M. C., Müller, M., and Gissmann, L.,** Antibodies to human papillomavirus and to other genital infectious agents and invasive cervical cancer risk. *Lancet* 341, 1116–1118, 1993.

69. **Lorinez, A. T., Reid, R., Jenson, A. B., Greenberg, M. D., Lancaster, W., and Kurman, R.,** Human papilloma virus infection of the cervix-relative risk association of 15 common anogenital types. *Obstet. Gynecol.* 79, 328–337, 1992.

70. **Rotking, I. D.,** Further studies in cervical cancer inheritance. *Cancer* 19, 1251–1268, 1966.
71. **Brinton, L. A., Tashima, K. T., Lehmann, H. F., Levine, R. S., Mallin, K., Savitz, D. A., Stolley, P. D., and Fraumeni, J. F.,** Epidemiology of cervical cancer by cell type. *Cancer Res.* 47, 1706–1711, 1987.
72. **Wank, R. and Thomssen, C.,** High risk of squamous cell carcinoma of the cervix for women with HLA-DQw3. *Nature* 352, 723–725, 1991.
73. **Apple, R. J. Erlich, H. A., Klitz, W., Manos, M. M., Becker, T. M., and Wheeler, C. M.,** HLA DR-DQ associations with cervical carcinoma show papillomavirus-type specificity. *Nat. Genet.* 6, 157–162, 1994.
74. **Hoskins, W. J., Perez, C. A., and Young, R. C.,** Gynecologic Tumors, In: *Cancer Principles & Practice of Oncology.* 4th Ed., De Vita, V. T., Jr., Hellman, S., and Rosenberg, S. A., Eds., J. B. Lippincott, Philadelphia, 1993, chap. 38.
75. **Sigurdsson, K.,** Effect of organized screening on the risk of cervical cancer. Evaluation of screening activity in Iceland, 1964–1991. *Int. J. Cancer* 54, 563–570, 1993.
76. **Goldgar, D. E., Easton, D. F., Cannon-Albright, L. A., and Skolnick, M. H.,** Systematic population-based assessment of cancer risk in first-degree relatives of cancer probands. *J. Natl. Cancer Inst.* 86, 1600–1608, 1994.
77. **Cannon-Albright, L. A., Thomas, A., Goldgar, D. E., Gholami, K., Rowe, K., Jacobsen, M., McWhorter, P., and Skolnick, M. H.,** Familiality of cancer in Utah. *Cancer Res.* 54, 2378–2385, 1994.
78. **Kemp, C. J., Wheldon, T., and Balmain, A.,** p53-Deficient mice are extremely susceptible to radiation-induced tumorigenesis. *Nat. Genet.* 8, 66–69, 1994.
79. **Khoury, M. J., Beaty, T. H., and Cohen, B. I., (Eds.),** *Fundamentals of Genetic Epidemiology,* Oxford University Press, New York, 1992.
80. **Morris, D. J. and Reis A.,** A YAC contig spanning the nevoid basal cell carcinoma syndrome, Fanconi anaemia group C, and xeroderma pigmentosum group A loci on chromosome 9q. *Genomics* 23, 23–29, 1994.

Chapter 3

THE PATHOLOGY OF GASTROINTESTINAL CANCER: CLUES TO FAMILIAL AGGREGATION

Grant N. Stemmermann

CONTENTS

I. INTRODUCTION

Familial clusters of cancer stem from shared environmental hazards, from a shared gene pool, or a combination of these. If a familial cancer trait is recognized, prophylactic intervention can eliminate an environmental hazard or soften the impact of a genetic defect, but a familial association may not be suspected if the index cancer is commonly encountered in the population at large.

Recognition of a familial cluster is most likely to occur if one of the affected relations has a tumor that displays some unusual features (e.g., onset before age 30), or when it involves an unusual primary site (e.g., small intestine, adrenal cortex). This chapter will focus on the primary sites of three common cancers — esophagus, stomach, and colorectum — and will put special emphasis upon family clusters that are commonly unrecognized rather than upon the classic, but uncommon, tumors that have well-established genetic origins (e.g., juvenile familial polyposis coli, Gardner syndrome, Peutz-Jeghers syndrome, etc.).

II. ESOPHAGUS

Squamous cell carcinoma is the most common esophageal malignancy and shows a strong male predominance. In Western Europe and North America it has been associated with alcoholism and heavy tobacco use.[1] These risk factors are usually not shared by an entire family and familial clusters of these tumors are not common. Improperly preserved food lacking in protective antioxidants characterize an environmental factor associated with squamous cancer in central Asia and China.[2] This diet, and its risks, is shared by the entire family. Segregation analysis indicates that an autosomal recessive Mendelian inheritance with a frequency of 19% causes 4% of these cancers in a high risk Chinese population.[2] Thus, both environmental and genetic esophageal cancer risk factors are combined in this population.

A less common autosomal dominant condition incurs almost certain development of squamous cell carcinoma of the esophagus. This trait is found in persons with late onset (i.e., 5–15 years of age) palmar and plantar hyperkeratosis.[3] Patients with this genetic defect develop carcinoma even though they abstain from alcohol or tobacco. The possibility of familial cancer should therefore be entertained when a careful medical history does not elicit evidence of these social habits. This possibility should certainly be considered if the patient is under 40 years of age and/or female.

Adenocarcinoma may arise in an area of dysplastic Barrett's metaplasia of the distal esophagus. This condition is associated with reflux esophagitis and gastric hyperacidity. It usually affects Caucasians and has a strong male predominance. The racial association suggests a genetic influence — an impression supported by observations of increased risk for synchronous asymptomatic colon cancer,[5] the occurrence of the tumor in identical twins,[6] and by one family cluster of these tumors.[7] The occurrence of the precursor lesion (Barrett's esophagus) in twin sisters offers additional support to this hypothesis.[8]

III. STOMACH

Cancer of the stomach appears in several different settings. Antral cancers predominate in populations exposed to the effects of *H. pylori* infection combined with a high salt diet deficient in antioxidant vitamins.[9] The infection is particularly common in poor children living in crowded housing.[10] The infection causes chronic gastritis (Figure 1) that persists throughout life, gradually evolving through several steps into intestinal metaplasia and carcinoma (Figure 2). Most of these tumors occur after 60 years of age. They are composed of neoplastic glands and form discrete metastasis to the liver and lungs. This form of stomach cancer has a strong tendency to occur in familial clusters because poor children in large families share its risk factors. Recognition of the concurrence of *H. pylori* infection and gastric cancer in an older man should alert the clinician to the possibility of similar gastritis and cancer risk among his siblings.

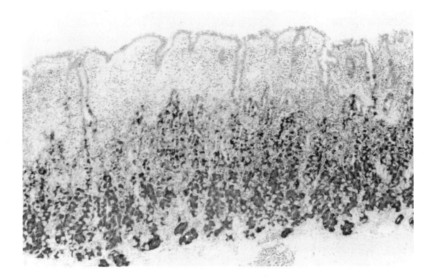

FIGURE 1. Superficial gastritis of corpus of the stomach due to *H. pylori* infection. The section shows infiltration of the lamina propria by dense collections of lymphocytes, plasma cells, and neutrophils. This change precedes atrophy. The chief cells are labeled with antibody against pepsinogen group II. (Hemotoxylin counter stain. × 40.)

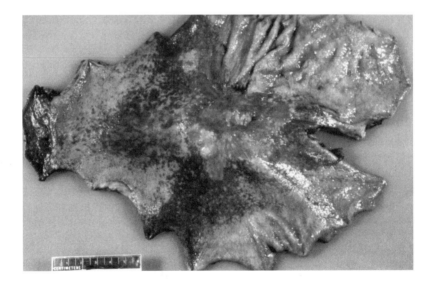

FIGURE 2. Gastric cancer on the lesser curvature of the stomach. The specimen has been stained to demonstrate alkaline phosphatase activity. This small gut enzyme is not normally found in the stomach. The cancer has developed at the site of maximal intestinal metaplasia on the lesser curvature near the junction of the antrum and corpus.

Cancer of the nonatrophic corpus may also be associated with *H. pylori* infection and superficial gastritis. These tumors are not preceded by intestinal metaplasia, have a diffuse growth pattern, and spread throughout the peritoneal cavity without forming discrete liver metastases (Figures 3 and 4). There is a suggestion of a genetic influence in the origin of this cancer since it tends to be the most common stomach cancer of young female patients (<45 years) and appears to show an association with blood type A.[11] Finnish studies indicate that familial gastric cancer is usually of the diffuse type and is especially common in women.[12] A recent Italian study also indicates a higher risk of familial cancer in female probands, but did not confirm the association with blood type A.[13]

Autoimmune, or type A, gastritis is associated with intestinal metaplasia, high serum gastrin levels, and autoantibodies against parietal cells. Patients with this disease have a high risk of acquiring gastric cancer, perhaps as a result of the trophic effects of gastrin upon both epithelial cells and fundic endocrine cells. The risk of acquiring this autoimmune disease is greatly increased among the first degree relatives of affected probands.[14] A highly specific marker for this type of gastritis is a serum pepsinogen group I (PG I) level below 20 ng/dl.[15]

Cancer of the cardia of the stomach arises in three distinct settings: (1) following partial gastrectomy for benign peptic ulcer, (2) in association with reflux esophagitis, and (3) as a manifestation of the hereditary non-polyposis syndrome (HNPCC). Only the last of these has a genetic basis which will be described in detail below. An example of the type of gastric cancer that may be encountered in this syndrome is shown in Figure 5. The index case had multicentric colon cancers and five of seven primary relatives with gastrointestinal cancer (Figure 6).

Sporadic adenomatous polyps of the stomach are much less common than those in the colon. Multiple adenomas are so uncommon that they constitute a strong indication of inherited risk and have been identified as a manifestation of familial colon polyposis.[16]

IV. SMALL INTESTINE

Adenomas and adenocarcinomas of the small intestine are very uncommon when compared to the stomach or large bowel. Familial clusters of carcinoma of the proximal small intestine have been associated with multicentric large bowel cancer and familial cancer clusters.[17] They probably represent examples of HNPCC. A multicenter study of familial adenomatous polyps has shown that 100 of 102 patients with this condition had duodenal adenomas and 11 had duodenal cancers of the ampullary region.[18] The proximal localization of these neoplasms in both HNPCC and FAP suggests an interaction between a genetic trait and mutagens in degraded bile salts. This concept is supported by the observation that the majority of small bowel cancers in a major cancer registry (Los Angeles) are found in the duodenum near the ampulla of Vater.[19]

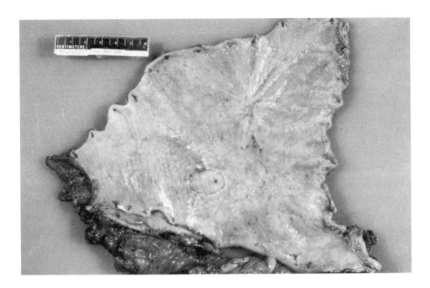

FIGURE 3. Diffuse gastric cancer arising in the nonintestinalized corpus. The specimen has been stained to demonstrate alkaline phosphatase. The enzyme is limited to the duodenum. Tumors of this type frequently arise in association with superficial gastritis similar to that shown in Figure 1.

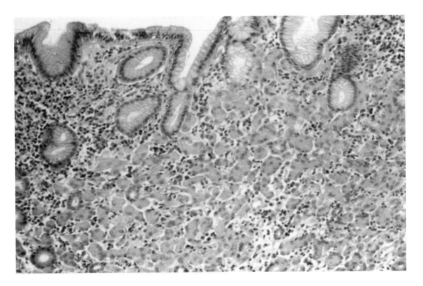

FIGURE 4. Microscopic appearance of the diffuse type tumor shown in Figure 3. There is no metaplasia. (H&E, × 40.)

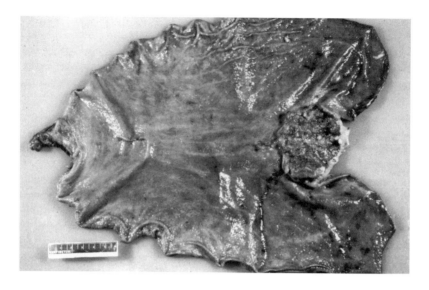

FIGURE 5. Adenocarcinoma of the cardia of the stomach in a patient with multicentric cancers and five of seven primary relatives with gastrointestinal cancer. The tumor measures 7 cm in diameter and is not associated with intestinal metaplasia. Despite its large size, the tumor was limited to the submucosa.

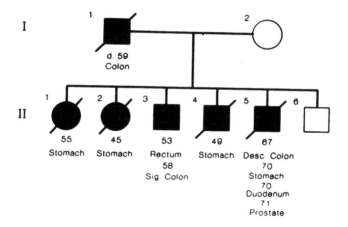

FIGURE 6. Kindred of the patient in Figure 5.

V. COLORECTUM

Large bowel cancer is the most common carcinoma affecting both sexes in North America, Western Europe, Australia, and New Zealand.[20] The dramatic increase in the frequency of this tumor among immigrants from low-risk Japan to high-risk U.S. indicates that environment plays a key role in its induction.[21]

In contrast, gastric carcinoma follows diametrically opposed trends in the frequency of gastric carcinoma.[21] Interestingly, members of families with multiple gastric carcinomas have higher rates of familial colon cancer than do other immigrants.[22] This suggests that inherited gene defects in these families render them vulnerable to environmental carcinogens specific to each tumor site.

Predisposition of some gastrointestinal tumors is clearly inherited. Adenomatous polyposis coli is a dominantly inherited disease with complete penetrance. When untreated, affected individuals will always develop carcinoma of the colorectum[23] or proximal small intestine.[18] Another inherited syndrome, HNPCC, is associated with an increased risk of colon cancer, usually involving the cecum, ascending colon, or proximal transverse colon.[24] Members of the affected families are also at high risk of developing cancers at sites other than the colon (e.g., breast, ovary, urothelium, stomach).[25]

HNPCC shows an autosomal dominant mode of inheritance, yet is characterized by a low, or incomplete, penetrance. Familial clusters of these cancer types are frequently not diagnosed as genetic because they involve sites that are commonly encountered in the population at large. The recent identification of genomic instability in a subset of colorectal cancers and the mapping of disease genes for *HNPCC* shows that inherited susceptibility to cancer can result from an inability to correct DNA mutations. At least two of the HNPCC genes (hMSH2 and hMLH3) are homologs of bacterial mismatch repair genes.[26-28] Germline mutations of p53, a gene known to function in response to DNA damage, also is associated with another cancer-prone disease known as the Li-Fraumeni syndrome.[29] These diseases suggest that subtle differences in the ability of an individual to respond to or repair DNA damage and errors of replication can influence an individual's risk of acquiring a cancer.

In the past, little attention has been paid to the possible role of environmental factors that might interact with genetic factors to induce gastrointestinal tumors. These interactions may explain the comparatively late age of onset of HNPCC tumors (55 years for colon carcinoma) as compared to APC tumors (34 years) and those that occur in the general population (65 years). They may also explain the multiorgan distribution of tumors in affected families and the frequent absence of tumors in some individuals who are obligate carriers of the mutant gene.

Recognition of the HNPCC syndrome depends on the diagnosis of cancer in a patient whose tumor meets the following criteria:[30] (1) three family members with colorectal cancer: (2) one of these must be a first-degree relative of the other two; (3) involvement of two generations; and (4) one patient must have developed large bowel cancer before 50 years of age. HNPCC is also associated with extracolonic malignancy,[25] and the definition may be extended to include tumor sites commonly associated with colorectal cancer in the same families: ovary, breast, small bowel, stomach, pancreas, bile duct, and urothelium.

Pending universal availability of molecular probes to identify high risk families, other clues to the presence of familial colorectal cancer should heighten the suspicion of inherited disease. For example: (1) the occurrence of multicentric cancers in the same person — these may be gastrointestinal, or may involve the ovary, breast, or urinary tract; (2) cancer of the proximal small intestine; and (3) large, diploid cancers of the right colon (i.e., a Dukes A cancer ≥ 10 cm in diameter).

VI. SUMMARY

In summary, the identification of familial clusters of cancer may also identify correctable environmental hazards or initiate screening programs to diagnose cancers at a treatable stage. The tumors and their precursors that should alert the physician to a possible family association are listed in Table 1.

TABLE 1
FAMILIAL GASTROINTESTINAL CANCER

Tumor site	Tumor type	Precursor	Environmental feature	Inherited feature
Esophagus	Squamous cell cancer	None	Undernutrition, malnutrition	Autosomal Mendelian inheritance
Esophagus	Squamous cell cancer	None	None	Tylosis, dominant Mendelian inheritance
Esophagus	Adenocarcinoma	Barrett's Metaplasia	Gastroesophageal reflux	None established but family clusters reported
Antrum stomach	Intestinal type	Chronic atrophic gastritis	*H. pylori* infection Malnutrition	None established but family clusters reported
Corpus stomach	Diffuse type	Superficial gastritis	*H. pylori* infection	Blood Type A
Cardia stomach	Intestinal type	None	None	HNPCC[1]
Small intestine	Adenocarcinoma	Adenoma	Degraded bile salts	HNPCC[1] FAP[2]
Right colon	Adenocarcinoma	Adenoma	Sedentary lifestyle Positive energy balance Low intake fiber antioxidant vitamins	HNPC[1] FAP[2]

[1]   HNPCC = Hereditary Non Polyposis Cancer Syndrome
[2]   FAP = Familial Adenomatous Polyposis

REFERENCES

1. **Day, N. E. and Munoz, N.,** Esophagus. In: *Cancer Epidemiology and Prevention*, Schottenfeld, D. and Fraumein, J., (Eds.) W. B. Saunders, Philadelphia, 1982, 596.
2. **Carter, C. L., Hu, N., and Wu, M.,** Segregation analysis of esophageal cancer in 221 high-risk Chinese families, *J. Natl. Cancer Inst.* 84, 771, 1992.
3. **McConnel, R. B.,** Single gene carcinoma of the Oesophagus. In: *The Genetics of Gastrointestinal Disorders.* Oxford Monographs on Medical Genetics, Oxford University Press, New York, 1966, 37.
4. **Sjogren, R. W. and Johnson, L. V.,** Barrett's esophagus: A review. *Am. J. Med.* 74, 313, 1983.
5. **Sonntag, S. J., Schnell, T. G., Chejfec, G., et al.** Barrett's oesophagus and colonic tumours. *Lancet* 1, 946, 1985.
6. **Gelfand, M. D.,** Barrett esophagus in sexagenarian twins. *J. Clin. Gastroenterol.* 5, 251, 1983.
7. **Everhart, C. W., Jr., Holzapple, P. G., and Humphries, T. J.,** Occurrence of Barrett's esophagus in three members of the same family. *Gastroenterology* 74, 1032(Abst.), 1978.
8. **Prior, A. and Whorwell, P. J.,** Familial Barrett's Oesophagus. *Hepatogastroenterology* 33, 86, 1956.
9. **Stemmermann, G. N.,** The role of *Helicobacter pylori* in the etiology of gastric cancer. In, *Cancer Prevention*, Devita, V. J., Hellmann, S., and Rosenberg, S. A., Eds., J. B. Lippincott, Philadelphia, 1991, 1.
10. **Correa, P., Fox, J., Fontham V. E., et al.,** *Helicobacter pylori* and gastric carcinoma. *Cancer* 66, 2569, 1990.
11. **Correa, P., Sasano, I., Stemmermann, G. N., and Haensel W.,** Pathology of gastric carcinoma in Japanese publications: Comparisons between Miyagi Prefecture, Japan and Hawaii. *JNCI*, 51–1449, 1973.
12. **Lehtola, J.,** Family study of gastric carcinoma: with special response to histologic types. *Scand. J. Gastroenterol.* 13 (Suppl. 50), 1–54, 1978.
13. **Palli, D., Galle, M., Caporas, N. E., Cipriani, F., DeCarli, A., Srieve, C., Fraumeni, J. F., and Buiatti, E.,** Family history and risk of stomach cancer, In, *Italy Cancer Epidemiol. Biomarkers Prev.* 3, 15, 1994.
14. **Varis, K., Samloff, I. M., Tiilikainen, A., Ihamaki, T., Kekki, M., Sipponen, P., and Siurala, M.,** Gastritis in first degree relatives of pernicious anemia, gastric cancer patients and controls. In: *The Genetics and Heterogeneity of Common Gastrointestinal Disorders*, Rotter, I., Samloff, I. M. and Remoin, D. L., Eds., Academic Press, New York, 1980, p 177.
15. **Samloff, I. M., Liebman, W. M., and Panitch, N. M.,** Serum group I pepsinogens by radioimmunoassay in control subjects and patients with peptic ulcer. *Gastroenterology* 69, 83, 1975.
16. **Utsunomiya, J., Maki, T., Iwama, T., Matsunaga, Y., Ichhikawa, T., Shimomura, T., Hamrgushi, E., and Aoki, N.,** Gastric lesion in familial polyposis coli. *Cancer* 34, 745, 1974.
17. **Stemmermann, G. N., Goodman, M. J., and Nomura, A. M. Y.,** Adenocarcinoma of the proximal small intestine. *Cancer* 70, 2766, 1992.
18. **Spigelman, A. D., Williams, C. B., Talbot, I. C., Domizio, P., and Phillips, R. K. S.,** Upper gastrointestinal cancer in patients with familial adenomatous polyposis. *Lancet* I, 783, 1989.
19. **Ross, R. K., Harnett, N. M., Bernstein, L., and Henderson, B. E.,** Epidemiology of adenocarcinoma of the small intestine: Is bile a bowel carcinogen? *Br. J. Cancer* 63, 143, 1991.
20. **Waterhouse, J., Muir, C., Shanmugaratnam, K., et al.,** Cancer incidence in five continents. Vol. IV, *IARC Publications,* Lyon, 1982.

21. **Stemmermann, G. N., Nomura, A. M. Y., and Kolonel, L. N.,** Cancer among Japanese in Hawaii. *Gann Monogr.* 33, 99, 1989.
22. **Stemmermann, G. N.,** Gastric cancer in Hawaiian Japanese: a familial study. In *Familial Cancer Control,* W. Weber et al., Eds., Springer-Verlag, Berlin, 1992, 23.
23. **Burt, R. W.,** Polyposis syndromes. In *Textbook of Gastroenterology* (Alpers, D. H., Owyang, C., Powell, D. W., and Silverstein, F. E., Eds.) J.P. Lippincott, Philadelphia, 1995, 1674.
24. **Lynch, H. T., Schuelke, G. S., Kimberling, W. J., Albano, W. A., Lynch, J., Biscone, K., Sanderg, A. A., Lipkin, M., Deschner, E. E., Mikol, Y. B., Elston, R. C., Bailey-Wilson, J., and Danes, B. S.,** Hereditary non polyposis colorectal cancer (Lynch I and II). *Cancer* 56, 939, 1985.
25. **Lynch, H. T., Richardson, J. D., Amin, M., Lynch, J., Cavalieri, R. J., Bronson, E., and Fusaro, R. M.,** Variable gastrointestinal and urologic cancers in a Lynch Syndrome II Kindred, *Dis. Colon Rectum* 34, 891, 1991.
26. **Leach, F. S., Nicolaides, N. C., Papadopoulos, N., Liu, B., Jin, J., Parsons, R., Peltomaki, P., Sipponen, P., Maltonen, L. A., and Vogelstein, B.,** Mutations of a mut S Homolog in hereditary non-polyposis colorectal cancer. *Cell* 75, 1215, 1993.
27. **Fishel, R., Lescoe, M. K., Rao, M. R. G., Copeland, N. G., Jenkins, N. A., Garber, J., Kane, M., and Kolodner, M.,** The human mutator gene MSH2 and its association with hereditary non-polyposis cancer syndrome. *Cell* 75, 1227, 1993.
28. **Parsons, R., Li, G. M., Longley, M. J., Fang, W. H., Papadopoulos, N., Jin, J., De La Chapelle, A., Kinzler, K. W., Vogelstein, B., and Modrich, P.,** Hypermutability and MIS Match Repair Deficiency in RER+ Tumor Cells. *Cell* 75, 1227, 1993.
29. **Malkin, D., Li, F. P., Strong, L. C., Fraumeni, J. R., Nelson, C. E., Kim, D. H., Kassel, J., Gryka, M. A., Bischoff, F. Z., Tainsky, M. A., and Friend, S. H.,** Germ-line p53 mutations in a familial syndrome of breast cancer, sarcoma and other neoplasms. *Science* 250, 1233, 1990.
30. **Vasen, H. P. A., Mecklin J. P., Meera Kahn, P., and Lynch, H. T.,** The international collaborative group on hereditary non-polyposis colorectal cancer (ICG-HNPCC) *Dis. Colon Rectum* 34, 424, 1991.

Chapter 4

FAMILIES WITH CANCER AT MULTIPLE SITES

Steven A. Narod

CONTENTS

I. INTRODUCTION

It is rare for the clinical geneticist to be faced with a pedigree which contains only one type of cancer. The majority of patients that present for clinical assessment of cancer risk describe a family history of cancer at multiple sites. Cancer is a very common condition, and almost all adults have at least one affected first- or second-degree relative. Furthermore, it now appears that the majority (if not all) of the genes which predispose carriers to cancer do so at more than one site. It is therefore important to inquire about all sites of cancer in relatives when evaluating a pedigree for the possibility of hereditary cancer. The clinician should be aware that members of families in which one site of cancer predominates may be at risk for cancers at additional sites; for example, it is prudent to offer ovarian cancer screening to women with familial breast cancer, and women in families with hereditary colon cancer should be advised of an increased risk of endometrial cancer.

II. METHODS OF STUDY

There are several analytic methods employed by genetic epidemiologists

0-8493-4782-3/96/$0.00+$.50

who wish to identify familial cancer syndromes and to establish the range of cancers featured in a particular syndrome. Case reports of large families have been fundamental in suggesting patterns. For example, in 1977 Chan and Pratt described a family with multiple cases of retinoblastoma, osteosarcoma, and cancer of the urinary tract.[1] It has since been determined by controlled follow-up studies that bladder cancer and osteosarcoma are increased in frequency in carriers of retinoblastoma mutations.

A cross-sectional observational study is a description of the number and sites of cancers in a series of pedigrees which are defined by a common feature. The distribution is compared to the expected distribution of cancers, based on surveys of the general population. Li and colleagues identified a panel of 24 families with tumors characteristic of the Li-Fraumeni syndrome.[2] A total of 191 neoplasms appeared in 151 family members — 30% of the tumors were soft tissue sarcomas, clearly in excess of expectations. However, these families were ascertained for sarcoma, and to some degree this excess was to be expected. Also, because cancer families come to our attention after several members are affected, it is likely that the extreme examples are the most closely studied. Because of this potential for referral bias, the optimal study design is to follow unaffected members of cancer families prospectively to estimate the rates and types of incident cancers. In this way, Garber et al. documented all new cases of cancer identified since the original 24 Li-Fraumeni families were ascertained, and were able to confirm the excess risk of sarcomas and breast cancers.[3] Unfortunately, few centers will have adequate numbers of families of sufficient size to perform this type of analysis.

Because of the difficulties in performing follow-up studies, most family cancer studies are either cross-sectional or case-control studies. The case-control study is the classic epidemiologic approach to studying the familial aggregation of cancer. The investigator must identify a series of cancer patients and healthy controls, and inquire about cancers in relatives of each group. Using the Iceland Tumor Registry, Tulinius et al. documented cancers in first- and second-degree relatives of 947 patients with breast cancer, and in spouse controls.[4] Increased risks were found for prostate cancer, for ovarian cancer, and for endometrial cancer. In another example, Schildkraut et al. found a relative risk of 3.6 for first-degree relatives and 2.9 for second-degree relatives with ovarian cancer in the CASH data base.[5]

An alternative approach is to perform segregation analysis. The goal of this statistical technique is to fit a genetic model (e.g., dominant, recessive, etc.) to a series of pedigrees, and to estimate the frequency and the penetrance of a predisposing gene in the population. A segregation analysis performed on a number of breast-ovarian cancer families led Lynch and colleagues to predict the existence of a dominant gene with a high lifetime penetrance of both breast and ovarian cancer.[6] The existence of this gene was later confirmed by linkage analysis.[7] In linkage analysis a particular genetic marker is found to segregate with the cancer susceptibility in the family; in the case of breast-ovarian cancer it was found that a marker on chromosome 17 was associated with breast or ovarian cancer in the great majority of women in three large families. This gene *(BRCA1)* has now been identified and appears to be involved in the regulation of gene transcription.[8]

Ultimately, when a cancer gene is identified, it becomes possible to survey families both for mutations and for cancer. The range of cancers associated with mutations of a susceptibility gene is then established and the clinical syndrome is better delineated.

In general, hereditary tumors cannot be distinguished from nonhereditary ones, and the diagnosis of familial cancer is made on historical grounds. However, one or more clues may alert the physician to the possibility that a cancer syndrome is present. Breast cancer appears at a much earlier age than expected in both the hereditary breast-ovarian[9] and Li-Fraumeni syndromes.[3] Hereditary colon and endometrial cancers are also of earlier onset than nonfamilial cases,[10] but the ages of onset of hereditary ovarian cancers are not remarkable.[11] Some tumor types may be associated with preneoplastic lesions in adjacent tissues; e.g., multiple polyposis associated with colon cancer is typical of familial adenomatous polyposis (FAP) and the presence of generalized C-cell hyperplasia in a patient with a medullary thyroid carcinoma is a signal that the patient may be from a family with multiple endocrine neoplasia. There is no convincing evidence yet that a preneoplastic lesion is associated with hereditary breast cancer, although atypical hyperplasia appears to be more frequent in families at increased risk.[12] The pathology of hereditary cancers may be different from their sporadic counterparts. Breast cancer of the medullary type is seen more commonly than expected in the breast-ovarian cancer syndrome and mucinous ovarian cancers are underrepresented.[13]

It has recently been shown that DNA from several of the forms of cancer associated with hereditary non-polyposis colon cancer (HNPCC) is prone to replication errors during mitosis and leads to the generation of new fragment sizes in polymorphic repeat sequences.[14] These tumor types include colon, rectum, pancreas, stomach, and endometrium. This phenomenon of microsatellite instability (the RER+ phenotype) is infrequent in sporadic tumors.[15] Replication errors appear to be more common in colon cancers which develop in young individuals — Lui and colleagues estimate that 58% of patients with colorectal cancer diagnosed before age 35 are associated with RER.[16] This laboratory technique may eventually prove to be useful to identify families which carry a high risk of cancer, but it cannot yet be used as an alternative to a careful family history. Up to 15% of colon cancers are associated with the RER phenomenon,[15] but the proportion of colon cancers associated with classical HNPCC is probably much smaller.

III. MULTISITE CANCER SYNDROMES

A. RETINOBLASTOMA

Retinoblastoma is an uncommon malignancy, representing about 3% of childhood cancers and affecting only 1 in 20,000 children (in contrast, breast cancer will affect 1 in 15 women before the age of 70). However, retinoblastoma is associated with the highest hereditary fraction of any cancer type, and it has been the subject of intensive study. Roughly 50% of children with retinoblastoma, including all those with bilateral disease, carry mutations in the retinoblastoma (*Rb1*) gene on chromosome 13q14. The retinoblastoma gene was one of the first hereditary cancer genes to be cloned and it has served as a model for other hereditary cancer syndromes. It is important that the family members of these cases be screened by ophthalmoscopy and by DNA analysis, because vision can often be preserved when tumors are diagnosed early.

Familial retinoblastoma was originally felt to be a site-specific form of hereditary cancer. One reason for this misconception is that the penetrance of the other tumor types associated with the *Rb1* gene is low, and with the exception of osteosarcoma, other cancers occur in adulthood. Survival has now improved to the point where patients can be followed for second cancers and it is apparent that carriers of *Rb1* mutations are at increased risk for osteosarcoma, brain tumors, melanoma, and cancers of the brain, bladder, lung, and pancreas.[17]

B. THE LI-FRAUMENI SYNDROME

The association of childhood sarcoma and adrenocortical cancer with early onset breast cancer, brain tumors, and leukemias (the Li-Fraumeni syndrome) has been mentioned above and is discussed elsewhere in this volume. There are no recognizable features which allow carriers of the susceptibility gene to be identified and the diagnosis is typically made on the basis of an unusual excess of cancer in the family. A large proportion of Li-Fraumeni families are associated with germline mutations of the p53 tumor suppressor gene.[18]

Garber et al. found 23 incident cancers in persons under age 45 in 24 Li-Fraumeni families, vs. 3.1 expected. Cancers seen in excess were sarcomas (3), breast (10), brain (4), leukemia (2), adrenocortical (1), and other (3). The incidence of breast cancer was 17.9 times higher than the incidence in the Connecticut Tumor Registry.[3] The highest relative risk, however, was for cancer of the adrenal cortex (relative risk = 111). Based on this extreme relative risk, it could be predicted that a high proportion of adrenal cortical tumors would be associated with the Li-Fraumeni syndrome. Recently, three of six children with this rare type of tumor were found to carry hereditary p53 mutations.[19] Similarly, Hartley et al. concluded that 5 of 151 children with soft-tissue sarcoma were from Li-Fraumeni families.[20]

C. MULTIPLE ENDOCRINE NEOPLASIAS

Multiple endocrine neoplasias (MEN) can be divided into two categories: those which affect the pituitary, parathyroid, and pancreas (MEN 1) and which are associated with an unidentified gene on chromosome 11, and those affecting primarily the thyroid C-cells and adrenal medulla (MEN 2) and which are associated with mutations in the *ret* proto-oncogene on chromosome 10q.[21] There are genetic variants of both types.

MEN 1 is characterized by hyperparathyroidism and by tumors of the pituitary (ACTH- and growth hormone-secreting tumors, prolactinomas) and the pancreatic islet cells. A variant of MEN 1 is characterized by a high frequency of carcinoid tumors and prolactinomas, and a low incidence of pancreatic tumors, and maps to the same chromosome 11 region.[22]

The consistent feature of MEN 2A is a dominant predisposition to medullary cancer of the thyroid. There is also a variable predisposition to pheochromocytoma; the extent of the pheochromocytoma risk is related to the particular site of the point mutation in the *ret* proto-oncogene.[21] A minority of families also have hyperparathyroidism. MEN 2B is the association of the same tumors with an unusual facial appearance (large lips, mucosal neuromas) and skeletal features resembling the Marfan syndrome. Approximately 25% of patients with medullary thyroid carcinoma are believed to be from families with a form of MEN 2.[23] In a recent study, 3 of 32 unselected patients with pheochromo-cytomas were found to be from MEN 2A families.[24] An additional 16 cases had von Hippel-Lindau disease.

D. BREAST-OVARIAN CANCER SYNDROMES

About 5% of breast and ovarian cancer cases are believed to be hereditary.[25,26] Families with breast and ovarian cancer have classically been divided into the Li-Fraumeni syndrome, hereditary site-specific breast cancer, the breast-ovarian cancer syndrome, site-specific ovarian cancer, and hereditary non-polyposis colon cancer.

With the advent of linkage analysis, the biological basis for distinguishing, or for merging, clinical subtypes has become better understood. A gene for early onset breast cancer, *BRCA1*, was mapped to chromosome 17q12 in 1990[27] and was identified in 1994.[8] *BRCA1* is responsible for the majority of families with multiple cases of breast and ovarian cancer, but for a minority of families with site-specific breast cancer.[28] On average, 85% of women with a *BRCA1* mutation will develop breast cancer and 45% will develop ovarian cancer by age 70.[29]

Among the common cancers, ovarian cancer is probably associated with the highest hereditary component. Between 3% and 7% of unselected women with ovarian cancer appear to be from families with hereditary predisposition.[26] With one affected first-degree relative, the lifetime risk of ovarian cancer rises from 1.4% to 5%. With two first-degree relatives affected the risk is approximately 30%. The hereditary fraction of breast cancer is probably slightly less than for ovarian cancer.[25] *BRCA1* mutations also appear to account for the majority of families with site-specific ovarian cancer.[30] The clinical distinction between the breast-ovarian cancer syndrome and site-specific ovarian cancer is not supported by recent linkage studies and it now seems likely that all women who carry *BRCA1* mutations are at risk for both breast and ovarian cancer. A large family[31] followed by Lynch and co-workers was found to be linked to the *BRCA1* in 1992, and the *BRCA1* mutation is now identified. At the time the genetic linkage study was completed there were ten documented cases of breast cancer and no ovarian cancers. The family was therefore classified as a site-specific breast cancer family. Recently, one of the carriers developed ovarian cancer. Another family was reported in the U.K. in which seven consecutive cases of ovarian cancer were followed by two early onset cases of breast cancer.[32]

It is possible that there will be different *BRCA1* mutations found to be associated with different penetrances of breast and ovarian cancer. Currently it is recommended that all carriers of *BRCA1* mutations be considered to be at risk for both cancer types. The majority of *BRCA1* mutations interrupt the genetic coding sequence and result in shortened (and presumably inactivated) protein.[33] Mutations have been observed over the length of the BRCA1 gene and several recurrent mutations have been identified. In these cases it appears that the shared mutations are inherited from common ancestors. For example, the majority of *BRCA1* mutations in Ashkenazi Jewish women are due to a single deletion of two nucleotides in codon 22,[34] and are associated with a common chromosome 17q haplotype.

In 1994, a second breast cancer susceptibility gene was mapped to chromosome 13q (*BRCA2*).[35] It now appears that the majority of large breast cancer families may be attributed to *BRCA1* and *BRCA2*. The clinical range of expression of *BRCA2* has not yet been clearly defined but it includes male breast cancer and prostate cancer.[36] The majority of families with cases of male breast cancer are linked to *BRCA2*.

E. COLON CANCER SYNDROMES

The traditional classification of the colon cancer syndromes has also been revised based on recent molecular findings. Families with florid adenomatous polyposis and those with an attenuated form of this disease (in which patients have fewer polyps) are both due to mutations in the *APC* gene.[37] Polyposis families are also at risk for stomach cancer and small intestinal malignancies, thyroid cancer, and hepatoblastoma. Some families are also at risk for brain tumors, in particular, childhood medulloblastoma (Turcot syndrome).[38] Watson and Lynch[10] et al. divided non-polyposis colon cancer into two clinical forms, depending on the presence of additional sites of cancer. Most HNPCC families are caused by mutations in either of two genes, one on chromosome 2 (*hMSH2*) and the other on chromosome 3 (*hMLH1*).[39,40] A few other families may be due to the *PMS1* and *PMS2* genes.[41] These four genes are involved in DNA mismatch repair. Mutations in these genes also predispose to cancer of the endometrium, the renal system, and possibly of the ovary. To date, no gene has been identified which appears to predispose to colon cancer in the absence of other forms of cancer. However, it remains possible that such a gene will be identified in the future.

IV. SCREENING FOR FAMILIAL CANCER

There are two fundamental steps in screening families at high risk of cancer. In the first step, families and individuals at increased risk are identified. Identification may be based on family history and clinical findings alone. It may be that all first-degree relatives of an affected individual are to be considered to be at high risk. For some diseases, preneoplastic lesions (e.g., adenomatous polyps in familial adenomatous polyposis (FAP), C-cell hyperplasia in multiple endocrine neoplasia (MEN 2A)) or other associated features (e.g., congenital hyperpigmentation of the retina in FAP, posterior cataracts in neurofibromatosis type 2 (NF2)) may suggest the carrier state. In addition, for several genetic cancer syndromes, specific DNA tests may be employed to identify family members who carry predisposing mutations.

The second step involves screening for the tumor itself in individuals found to be at genetic risk. Some of the recommended screening tests (e.g., mammography) are in conventional use; others (e.g., pentagastrin-stimulated calcitonin levels in MEN 2A) are specific for persons with genetic conditions.

Because the presence of a predisposing cancer mutation cannot be inferred purely on clinical or histologic grounds, the molecular geneticist must examine the DNA. There are currently two approaches to molecular diagnosis. If the sequence of a susceptibility gene is known in its normal and mutant forms, then a mutation can be sought directly in the DNA taken from lymphocytes in the blood. This technique is often called the direct method, in contrast to linkage analysis in which a statistical association is sought between a genetic marker and the clinical appearance of cancer in several related individuals.

It is hoped that presymptomatic detection of carriers using DNA testing will permit screening efforts to concentrate on those individuals at highest risk. In many situations, DNA analysis will permit the majority of the individuals in the family who are believed to be at risk to be excluded from further investigation. For example, 82 individuals in 13 families with neurofibromatosis type 2 (NF2) were considered to be at risk for developing acoustic neuromas and meningiomas prior to genetic testing.[42] By using chromosome 22 linked markers it was possible to effectively rule out the NF2 carrier state for 65% of these. The 13 individuals (16%) who were found to be at high risk for the disease could be offered more intensive screening. When the NF2 gene was cloned, it became possible to do direct screening of DNA for mutations. Because of the relatively large size of the NF2 gene (17 exons) DNA is often screened for abnormal banding patterns with single-strand conformational analysis (SSC) before sequencing is done. Using this two-step process, it was possible to identify mutations in 60% of 58 unrelated individuals with NF2.

Many oncology centers in the U.S. are now developing programs in predictive testing for cancer. These include geneticists and genetic counsellors in their management teams. Family cancer clinics have arisen to meet the demand of patients and physicians and to apply our evolving knowledge of the genetic map to the prevention and management of hereditary cancer. The practice of genetic medicine differs from conventional medicine in several important ways: for the geneticist the basic unit of observation is the family, but the patient-doctor relationship extends to only the individual seeking advice. Because clinical information on all related family members is relevant to the evaluation, the genetic analysis of families is complex and requires an ongoing commitment to the families to assimilate new information and to advise them appropriately.

Once carriers of predisposing mutations are identified, our attention turns toward the prevention and early detection of cancers in the individuals found to be at risk. For several cancer syndromes the relative merits of prophylactic surgery and intensified screening must be considered. For example, young adults found to carry a gene mutation in the *ret* oncogene, which predisposes to medullary cancer of the thyroid in the context of multiple endocrine neoplasia type 2 (MEN 2A), may be followed by annual screening using the pentagastrin stimulation test[43,44] or may opt for prophylactic thyroidectomy.

Women who are believed to carry mutations of the *BRCA1* gene are at high risk for ovarian cancer.[29] The benefits and limitations of ovarian cancer screening should be discussed with the woman and compared with prophylactic oophorectomy. There is currently much interest in evaluating ovarian ultrasound in screening for ovarian cancer. Using transvaginal ultrasound with color flow imaging, Weiner et al.[45] found ovarian cancer in 4 of 600 women with a past history of breast cancer (this group is at roughly double the risk of ovarian cancer as is the general public). Muto et al.[46] screened 386 women with a family history of ovarian cancer using transvaginal sonography, color flow Doppler and CA-125. The ultrasound examination was abnormal in 23% of the women, but no malignant ovarian lesion was detected. Bourne et al.[47] identified 3 cases of stage Ia ovarian cancer in 776 women with a family history of ovarian cancer. Because of the high lifetime risk of ovarian cancer associated with *BRCA1*, and because the sensitivity and effectiveness of the current methods of screening are uncertain, groups currently recommend prophylactic removal of the ovaries of *BRCA1* carriers around the time of menopause.[48] Unfortunately, up to 5% of these women will later develop peritoneal cancer.[49]

The role of prophylactic mastectomy in hereditary breast cancer is more controversial. There is currently little evidence that screening of young women by mammography will reduce the mortality from breast cancer. It has not yet been possible to address this question specifically in women at high familial risk, but there is little reason to believe that sensitivity of the mammography is better or the natural history of breast cancer is different in women at high familial risk. There have been rare cases of breast cancer among women who have undergone prophylactic removal of the breasts.

While it is currently accepted that preventive colectomy reduces mortality for adults with FAP, the relative value of screening vs. prophylactic surgery for carriers of genes for HNPCC has not yet been established. There is good evidence that sigmoidoscopy is beneficial in reducing mortality from cancer of the rectum and the distal colon[50] and that colonoscopy, followed by polypectomy when indicated, reduces the incidence of invasive colon cancer.[51] Colonoscopy is currently recommended from an early age in HNPCC families, but it should be noted that the natural history of hereditary colon cancer may differ from sporadic cancer. Hereditary colon cancer is usually right-sided and beyond the reach of the sigmoidoscope. Furthermore, it has not been established if colon cancers in HNPCC families occur in preexisting polyps.[52,53] It will be of primary importance to establish the relative benefits of screening vs. prophylactic surgery in individuals who carry HNPCC gene mutations.

REFERENCES

1. **Chan, H. and Pratt, C. B.** A new familial cancer syndrome? A spectrum of malignant and benign tumors including retinoblastoma, carcinoma of the bladder and other genitourinary tumours, thyroid adenoma and a probable case of multifocal osteosarcoma. *J. Natl. Cancer Inst.*, 58, 205, 1977.
2. **Li, F. P., Fraumeni, J. F., Mulvihill, J. J., Blattner, W. A., Dreyfus, M. G, Tucker, M. A., and Miller, R. W.** A cancer family syndrome in twenty-four kindreds. *Cancer Res.*, 48, 5358, 1988.
3. **Garber, J. E., Goldstein, A. M., Kantor, A. F., Dreyfus, M. G., Fraumeni, J. F., and Li, F. P.** Follow up study of twenty-four families with the Li-Fraumeni syndrome. *Cancer Res.*, 51, 6094, 1991.
4. **Tulinius, H., Egilsson, V., Olafsdottir, G. H., and Sigvaldason, H.** Risk of prostate, ovarian and endometrial cancer among relatives of women with breast cancer. *Br. Med. J.*, 305, 855, 1992.
5. **Schildkraut, J. M., Risch, N., and Thompson, W. D.** Evaluating genetic association among ovarian, breast, and endometrial cancer: evidence for a breast/ovarian cancer relationship. *Am. J. Hum. Genet.*, 45, 521–529, 1989.
6. **Go, R. C. P., King, M. C., Bailey-Wilson, J., Elston, R. C., and Lynch, H. T.** Genetic epidemiology of breast cancer and associated cancers in high-risk families. I. Segregation analysis. *J. Natl. Cancer Inst.*, 71, 455, 1983.
7. **Narod, S. A., Feunteun, J., Lynch, H., Watson, P., Conway, T., Lynch, J., and Lenoir, G. M.** A familial breast-ovarian cancer locus on chromosome 17q12-23. *Lancet*, 338, 82, 1991.
8. **Miki, Y., Swansen, J., Shattuck-Eidens, D., Futreal, F. A., Harshman, K., Tavrigan, S., Lui, Q., Cochran, C., Brennen, L. M., Ding, W., Bell, R., Rosenthal, J., Hussey, C., Tran, T., McClure, M., Frye, C., Harder, T., Phelps, R., Haugen-Strano, A., Katcher, H., Yakumo, K., Gholarni, Z., Shaffer, D., Stone, S., Bayer, S., Wray, C., Bogden, R., Dayanath, P., Ward, J., Tonin, P., Narod, S. A., Bristow, P. K., Norris, F. H., Helvering, L., Morrison, P., Rosteck, P., Lai, M., Barrett, J. C., Lewis, C., Neuhausen, S., Cannon-Albright, L., Goldgar, D., Wiseman, R., Kamb, A., and Skolnick, M. H.** A strong candidate for the breast and ovarian cancer susceptibility gene, BRCA1. *Science*, 266, 66, 1994.

9. **Claus, E. B., Risch, N., and Thompson, W. D.** Age of onset as an indicator of familial risk of breast cancer. *Am. J. Epidemiol.*, 131, 961, 1990.

10. **Watson, P. and Lynch, H. T.** Extracolonic cancer in hereditary nonpolyposis colorectal cancer. *Cancer*, 71, 677, 1993.

11. **Amos, C. I., Shaw, G. L., Tucker, M. A., and Hartge, P.** Age at onset for familial epithelial ovarian cancer. *J. Am. Med. Assoc.*, 268, 1896, 1992.

12. **Dupont, W. D. and Page, D. L.** Breast cancer risk associated with proliferative disease, age at first birth and a family history of breast cancer. *Am. J. Epidemiol.*, 125, 769, 1987.

13. **Narod, S. A., Tonin, P., Lynch, H. T., Watson, P., Feunteun, J., and Lenoir, G. M.** Histology of BRCA1-associated ovarian tumours. *Lancet*, 343, 236, 1994.

14. **Thibodeau, S. N., Bren, G., and Schaid D.** Microsatellite instability in cancer of the proximal colon. *Science*, 260, 816–819, 1993.

15. **Lothe, R. A., Peltomaki, P., Meling, G. I., Aaltonen, L. A., Nystrom-Lahti, M., Pylkkanen, L., Heimdal, G., Anderson, T. I., Moller, P., Rognum, T. O., Fossa, S. D., Hadorsen, T., Langmark, F., Brogger, A., de la Chapelle, A., and Borresen, A.-L.** Genomic instability in colorectal cancer: relationship to clinicopathological variables and family history. *Cancer Res.*, 53, 5489, 1993.

16. **Lui, B., Farrington, S. M., Petersen, G. M., Hamilton, S. R., Parsons, R., Papadopolous, N., Fujiwara, T., Jen, J., Kinzler, K. W., Wyllie, A. H., Vogelstein, B., and Dunlop, M. G.** Genetic instability occurs in the majority of young patients with colorectal cancer. *Nat. Med.*, 4, 348, 1995.

17. **Eng, C., Li, F. P., Abramson, D. H., Ellsworth, R. M., Wong, F. L., Goldman, M. B., Seddon, J., Tarbell, N., and Boice, J. D.** Mortality from second tumors among long-term survivors of retinoblastoma. *J. Natl. Cancer Inst.*, 85, 1121, 1993.

18. **Malkin, D., Li, F. P., Strong, L. C., Fraumeni, J. F., Nelson, C. E., Kim, D. H., Kassel, J., Gryka, M. A., Bischoff, F. Z., Tainsky, M. A., and Friend, S. H.** Germ line p53 mutations in a familial syndrome of breast cancer, sarcomas and other neoplasms. *Science*, 250, 1233, 1990.

19. **Wagner, J., Portwine, C., Rabin, K., Leclerc, J.-M., Narod, S. A., and Malkin, D.** A high frequency of germline mutations in childhood adrenocortical cancer. *J. Natl. Cancer Inst.*, 86, 1707, 1994.

20. **Hartley, A. L., Birch, J. M., Blair, V., Kelsey, A. M., Harris, M., Morris, M., and Jones, P. H.** Patterns of cancer in the families of children with soft tissue sarcoma. *Cancer*, 72, 923, 1993.

21. **Mulligan, L. M., Eng, C., Healey, C. S., Clayton, D., Kwok, J. B. J., Gardner, E., Ponder, M. A., Frilling, A., Jackson, C. E., Lehnert, H., Neumann, H. P. H., Thibodeau, S. N., and Ponder, B. A. J.** Specific mutations of the RET proto-oncogene are related to disease phenotype in MEN2A and FMTC. *Nat. Genet.*, 6, 70, 1994.

22. **Petty, E. M., Green, J. S., Marx, S. J., Taggart, R. T., Farid, N., and Bale, A. E.** Mapping the gene for hereditary hyperparathyroidism and prolactinoma (MEN1 Burin) to chromosome 11q: evidence for a founder effect in patients from Newfoundland. *Am. J. Hum. Genet.*, 54, 1060, 1994.

23. **Saad, R. K., Ordonez, N. G., Rashid, R. K., Guido, J. J., Stratton-Hill, C., Hickey, R. C., and Samaan, N. A.** Medullary carcinoma of the thyroid. A study of the clinical features and prognostic factors in 161 patients. *Medicine*, 63, 319, 1984.

24. **Neumann, H. P. H., Berger, D. P., Sigmund, G., Blum, U., Schmidt, D., Parmer, R. J. H., Volk, B., and Kirset, G.** Pheochromocytomas, multiple endocrine neoplasia type 2 and Von Hippel-Lindau disease. *N. Engl. J. Med.*, 329, 1531, 1993.

25. **Lynch, H. T. and Lynch J. F.** Breast cancer in an oncology clinic: 328 consecutive patients. *Cancer Genet. Cytogenet.*, 23, 369, 1986.

26. **Narod, S. A., Madlensky, L., Bradley, L., Cole, D., Tonin, P., Rosen, B., and Risch, H.** Hereditary and familial ovarian cancer in Southern Ontario. *Cancer*, 74, 2341, 1994.

27. **Hall, J. M., Lee, M. K., Newman, B., Morrow, J. E., Anderson, L. A., Huey, B., and King, M.-C.** Linkage of early-onset familial breast cancer to chromosome 17q21. *Science*, 250, 1684, 1990.
28. **Narod, S. A., Ford, D., Devilee, P., Barkardottir, R., Lynch, H. T., Smith, S. A., Ponder, B. A. J., Weber, B. L., Garber, J., Birch, J. M., Cornelis, R. S., Kelsell, D. P., Spurr, N., Smyth, E., Haites, N., Sobol, H., Bignon, Y. J., Claude-Chang, J., Hamann, U., Lindblom, A., Borg, A., Piver, M. S., Gallion, H. H., Struewing, J., Whittemore, A., Tonin, P., Goldgar, D., Easton, D. F., and the Breast Cancer Linkage Consortium.** An evaluation of genetic heterogeneity in 145 breast-ovarian cancer families. *Am. J. Hum. Genet.*, 56, 254, 1995.
29. **Ford, D., Easton, D. F., Bishop, D. T., Narod, S. A., and Goldgar, D. E.** The risks of cancer in BRCA1 mutation carriers. *Lancet* 343, 692, 1994.
30. **Steichen-Gersdorf, E., Gallion, H. H., Ford, D., Girodet, C., Easton, D. F., DiCioccio, R. A., Evans, G., Ponder, M. A., Pye, C., Mazoyer, S., Noguchi, T., Karengueven, F., Sobol, H., Hardouin, A., Bignon, Y.-J., Piver, M. S., Smith, S. A., and Ponder, B. A. J.** Familial site-specific ovarian cancer is linked to BRCA1 on 17q12-21. *Am. J. Hum. Genet.*, 55, 870, 1994.
31. **Tonin, P., Serova, O., Simard, J., Lenoir, G., Feunteun, J., Morgan, K., Lynch, H. T., and Narod, S. A.** The gene for hereditary breast cancer, BRCA1, maps distal to EDH17B2 in chromosome region 17q12-q21. *Hum. Mol. Genet.*, 3, 1679, 1994.
32. **Evans, D. G. R, Ribiero, G., Warrell, D., and Donnai, D.** Ovarian cancer family and prophylactic choices. *J. Med. Genet.*, 29, 416, 1992.
33. **Shattuck-Eidens D., MacLure, M., Simard, J., Labrie, F., Narod, S. A., Weber, B., Collins, F., Friedman, L., Ostermeyer, E., Szabo, C., King, M. C., Jhanwar, S., Offit, K., Norton, L., Gilewski, T., Lubin, M., Osborne, M., Black, D., Boyd, M., Steel, M., Ingles, S., Haile, R., Borg, A., Lindblom, A., Gayther, S., Ponder, B., Warren, B., Stratton, M., Qingyun, L., Kamb, A., Fujimura, F., Skolnick, M., and Goldgar, D.** Collaborative survey of 82 mutations in the BRCA1 breast and ovarian cancer susceptibility gene. *J. Am. Med. Assoc.*, 273, 535, 1994.
34. **Tonin, P., Serova, O., Lenoir, G., Lynch, H., Durocher, F., Simard, J., Morgan, K., and Narod, S. A.** BRCA1 mutations in Ashkenazi Jewish women. *Am. J. Hum. Genet.*, 57, 189, 1995.
35. **Wooster, R., Neuhausen, S., Mangion, J., Quirk, Y., Ford, D., Collins, N., Nguyen, K., Seal, S., Tran, T., Averill, D., Fields, P., Marshall, G., Narod, S. A., Lenoir, G. M., Lynch, H. T., Devilee, P., Cornelisse, C. J., Menko, F. H., Daly, P. A., Ormiston, W., McManus R., Pye C., Cannon-Albright, L., Peto, J., Ponder, B. A. J., Skolnick, M., Easton, D. E., Goldgar, D. E., and Stratton, M. R.** Localisation of a breast cancer susceptibility gene (BRCA2) to chromosome 13q by genetic linkage analysis. *Science*, 265, 2088, 1994.
36. **Tonin, P., Ghadirian, P., Phelan, C., Lenoir, G., Lynch, H., and Narod, S. A.** A large multisite cancer family is linked to BRCA2. *J. Med. Genet.*, in press.
37. **Spirio, L., Olschwang, S., Groden, J., Robertson, M., Samowitz, W., Joslyn, G., Gelbert, L., Thilveris, A., Carlson, M., Otterud, B., Lynch, H., Watson, P., Lynch, P., Laurent-Puig, P., Burt, R., Hughers, J. P., Thomas, G., Leppert, M., and White, R.** Alleles of the APC gene. An attenuated form of familial polyposis. *Cell*, 75, 951, 1993.
38. **Hamilton, S. R., Liu, B., Parsons, R. E., Papadopolous N., Jen, J., Powell, S. M., Krush, A. J., Berk, T., Cohen, Z., Tetu, B., Burger, P. C., Wood, P. A., Taqi, F., Booker, S. V., Petersen, G. M., Offerhaus, G. J. A., Tersmette, A. C., Giardiello, F. M., Vogelstein, B., and Kinzler, K. K.** The molecular basis of Turcot's syndrome. *N. Engl. J. Med.*, 332, 839, 1995.
39. **Fishel, R., Lescoe, M. K., Rao, M. R. S., Copeland, N. G., Jenkins, N. A., Garber, J., Kane, M., and Kolodner, R.** The human mutator gene homolog MSH2 and its association with hereditary nonpolyposis colon cancer. *Cell*, 75, 1027, 1993.

40. Bronner, C. E., Baker, S. M., Morrison, P. T., Warren, G., Smith, L., Lescoe, M. K., Kane, M., Earabino, C., Lipford, J., Lindblom, A., Tannergard, P., Bollag, R. J., Godwin, A. R., Ward, D. C., Nordenskjold, M., Fishel, R., Kolodner, R., and Liskay, R. M. Mutation in the DNA mismatch repair gene homologue hMLH1 is associated with hereditary non-polyposis colon cancer. *Nature*, 368, 258, 1994.

41. Nicolaides, N. C., Papadopolous, N., Lui, B., Wei, Y.-F., Carter, K. C., Ruben, S. M., Rosen, C. A., Haseltine, W. A., Fleischmann, R. C., Fraser, C. M., Adams, M. D., Venter, J. C., Dunlop, M. G., Hamilton, S. R., Petersen, G. M., de la Chapelle, A., Vogelstein, B., and Kinzler, K. W. Mutations of two PMS homologues in hereditary non-polyposis colon cancer. *Nature*, 371, 75, 1994.

42. Ruttledge, M. H., Narod, S. A., Dumanski, J. P., Parry, D. M., Eldridge, R., Wertelecki, W., Parboosingh, J., Faucher, M.-C., Lenoir, G. M., Collins, V. P., Nordenskjold, M., and Rouleau, G. A. Pre-symptomatic diagnosis for neurofibromatosis type 2 employing a combination of chromosome 22 markers. *Neurology*, 43, 1753, 1993.

43. Gagel, R. F., Tashjian, A. H., Cummings, T., Papathanasopolous, N., Kaplan, M. M., DeLellis, R. A., Wolfe, R. J., and Reichlin, S. Clinical outcome of prospective screening for multiple endocrine neoplasia type 2a. *N. Engl. J. Med.*, 318, 478, 1988.

44. Lips, C. J. M., Landsvater, R. M., Hoppener, J. W. M., Geerdink, R. A., Blijham, G., Van Gils, A. P. G., De Witt, M. J., Zewald, R. A., Berends, M. J. H., Beemer, F. M., Jansen, R. P. M., Van Amstel, H. K. P., Van Vroonhoven, T. J. M. V., and Vroom, T. M. Clinical screening as compared with DNA analysis in families with multiple endocrine neoplasia type 2a. *N. Engl. J. Med.*, 331, 828, 1994.

45. Weiner, Z., Beck, D., Shteiner, M., Borovick, R., Ben-Shachar, M., Robinzon, E., and Brandes, J. M. Screening for ovarian cancer in women with breast cancer and transvaginal sonography and color flow imaging. *J. Ultrasound Med.*, 12, 387, 1993.

46. Muto, M. G., Cramer, D. W., and Brown, D. L. Screening for ovarian cancer: the preliminary experience of a familial ovarian cancer center. *Gynecol. Oncol.*, 51, 12, 1993.

47. Bourne, T. H., Whitehead, M. I., Campbell, S., Royston, P., Bhan, V., and Collins, W. P. Ultrasound screening for ovarian cancer. *Gynecol. Oncol.*, 43, 92, 1991.

48. Kerlikowske, K., Brown, J. S., and Grady, D. G. Should women with familial ovarian undergo prophylactic oophorectomy?, *Obstet. Gynecol.*, 80, 700, 1992.

49. Tobacman, J. K., Tucker, M. A., Kase, R., Greene, M., Costa, J., and Fraumeni, J. F. Intra-abdominal carcinomatosis after prophylactic oophorectomy in ovarian cancer prone families. *Lancet*, 2, 795, 1982.

50. Selby, J. V., Friedman, G. D., Quesenberry, C. P., and Weiss, N. S. A case-control study of screening sigmoidoscopy and mortality from colorectal cancer. *N. Engl. J. Med.*, 326, 653, 1992.

51. Winawer, S. J., Zauber, A. G., Ho, M. N., O'Brien, M. J., Gottleib, L. S., Sternberg, S. S., Waye, J. D., Schapiro, M., Bond, J. H., Panish, J. F., Ackroyd, F., Shike, M., Kurtz, R. C., Hornsby-Lewis, L., Gerdes, H., Steward, E. T., and the National Polyp Study Workshop, et al. Prevention of colorectal cancer by colonosocopic polypectomy. *N. Engl. J. Med.*, 329, 1977, 1993.

52. Jass, J. R., Stewart, S. M., Stewart, J., and Lane, M. R. Hereditary non-polyposis colorectal cancer — morphologies, genes and mutations. *Mutat. Res.*, 310, 125, 1994.

53. Vasen, H. F. A., Nagengast, F. M., and Khan, P. M. Interval cancers in hereditary non-polyposis colorectal cancer (Lynch syndrome). *Lancet*, 345, 1183, 1985.

Chapter 5

THE LI-FRAUMENI SYNDROME

David Malkin

CONTENTS

I. INTRODUCTION

Virtually every type of cancer has been reported to occur in a familial form, and several single-gene disorders are associated with an excessively high risk of cancer. Studies of these hereditary cancer clusters have led to the identification of genes found to be critical to both carcinogenesis and normal human development. Some of these conditions, including the multiple endocrine neoplasias, neurofibromatoses, von Hippel-Lindau disease, and Gorlin syndrome (nevoid basal cell carcinoma syndrome) are represented primarily by the development of cancer, whereas in others, such as ataxia-telangiectasia, Bloom syndrome, and Fanconi anemia, cancer appears in association with nonmalignant manifestations. The Li-Fraumeni syndrome (LFS) is a rare, yet important familial cancer syndrome. The wide spectrum of neoplasms found in LFS families, the early onset of disease, the tendency to develop multiple primary tumors, and the association of germline mutations of a critical growth-regulatory gene (p53), contribute to our understanding of malignant disease.

0-8493-4782-3/96/$0.00+$.50
© 1996 by CRC Press Inc.

Problems arising from the identification of a cancer-predisposing gene in LFS and the potential for predictive genetic testing for cancer risk introduce complex issues of the psychosocial, ethical, and legal impact on families and society at large. This chapter describes the clinical presentation of LFS and presents evidence which implicates the *p53* tumor suppressor gene in the development of cancer in these families. The problems of genetic heterogeneity and the potential impact of predictive genetic testing for this multicancer disorder are addressed.

II. THE LI-FRAUMENI SYNDROME

The results of a retrospective survey of over 600 medical records, death certificates, and family histories of children with rhabdomyosarcoma diagnosed in the U.S. were reported by Li and Fraumeni in 1969.[1,2] In five families, siblings or cousins of the proband had also developed a childhood sarcoma. On the ancestral line of one parent in each family diverse cancers of distinct histopathologies were observed to occur at a frequency much greater than expected. Breast carcinoma in female relatives and soft-tissue sarcomas were most commonly represented. Acute leukemias, brain tumors, carcinomas of the lung, pancreas, and skin in first- and second-degree relatives, and adrenocortical carcinomas in siblings of the proband were also observed in excess. Subsequent prospective analysis of similarly affected families has refined the list of cancers in affected members from the originally described soft tissue sarcomas and breast cancer to now include osteosarcoma, brain tumors, leukemias, and adrenocortical carcinoma.[3-5] This family cancer syndrome is known as the Li-Fraumeni syndrome and is represented by the "classic" pedigree shown in Figure 1 and Table 1. The familial occurrence of neoplasms of discordant histopathologic sites was initially considered to be phenotypically equivalent to the occurrence of multiple primary tumors in a single individual.[1] Epidemiologic studies have confirmed that neoplasms in LFS families tend to occur in children and young adults, often as multiple primary cancers.[3,4] Although other hereditary cancer disorders, such as neurofibromatosis and Beckwith-Wiedemann syndrome are characterized by the occurrence of tumors at unusually early ages and at multiple sites, the constellation of tumors is distinct.

The observed cancer distribution in LFS best fits a rare autosomal dominant gene model of inheritance.[6] The probability of developing any invasive malignancy (excluding skin cancer) approaches 50% by age 30, at which age only 1% of the general population has developed cancer. More than 90% of gene carriers are predicted to develop cancer by age 70. On careful examination, it appears that the age of onset of tumors frequently decreases with each subsequent generation.[3] Whether this phenomenon of "anticipation" results from ascertainment bias or from some as yet undetermined genetic or epigenetic phenomenon is not known.

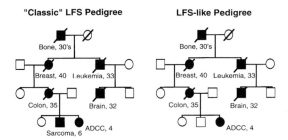

FIGURE 1. Comparison between a "classic" Li-Fraumeni syndrome pedigree (left panel) in which the proband is diagnosed with sarcoma at age 6 and has two first-degree relatives (sister with adrenocortical carcinoma and mother with colon cancer) diagnosed before age 45. Multiple other family members along the maternal line are affected. The pedigree on the right side is similar, except that there is no sarcoma patient. Although the woman with colon cancer has two first-degree relatives with cancer (mother with breast cancer and daughter with adrenocortical carcinoma), the family represents an incomplete or LFS-like pedigree.

TABLE 1
Relative Frequency of Component and Possible Tumor Types in 24 Li-Fraumeni Syndrome Families

Tumor type	Age at Diagnosis (years)			All Ages
	0–14	15–49	>44	
Component tumors of LFS				
Breast carcinoma	0	49	11	60
Soft tissue sarcoma	13	12	4	29
Brain tumors	12	15	1	28
Osteosarcoma	6	6	2	14
Leukemia	8	4	2	14
Adrenocortical cancer	5	0	0	5
Possible component tumors				
Lung carcinoma	0	7	12	19
Prostate carcinoma	0	0	8	8
Pancreas carcinoma	0	1	6	7
Melanoma	0	1	2	3
Other cancers	6	24	14	44
All cancers	50	119	62	231

Note: All families were ascertained through a proband with sarcoma, who is excluded from the tabulations.

Adapted from Garber, J.E., Goldstein, A.M., Kantor, A.F., et al., *Cancer Res.*, 51, 6094–6097, 1991. With permission.

The potential for ascertainment bias has complicated the interpretation of the original description and subsequent characterization of LFS families. One prospective study[4] suggests that bias may arise from the preferential selection of the most dramatically affected kindreds or the possibility of chance association of cancers in rare families. Other problems include the inability to accurately determine the prevalence of the syndrome in the general population, and uncertainties in defining both the spectrum of cancers in the syndrome and the penetrance of the predisposing gene(s). Nevertheless, this study monitored 24 LFS families over many years, and revealed continued expression of the dominantly inherited syndrome among young family members.[4] Cancer excesses were confined to the six previously described sites. The "classic" definition of LFS requires one individual (usually the proband) to be diagnosed with a sarcoma before 45 years of age, a first-degree relative with cancer before 45 years of age, and another first- or second-degree relative in the same parental lineage with any cancer diagnosed under 45, or with sarcoma at any age.[4] Clearly, the identification of a defective gene or genes conferring cancer predisposition in these families would assist in refining the definition of the syndrome.

Early laboratory studies to determine genetic factors implicated in LFS were subject to several limitations. The mortality rate among affected family members was high, and available tissues and blood samples were few. Cancers occurring in relatives who were not gene carriers, or *phenocopies*, could not be distinguished from cancers in gene carriers. Non-random constitutional karyotypic alterations were not found in affected family members. Associated phenotypic malformations are not seen in LFS families, and therefore the LFS gene(s) could not be mapped in the same fashion that the presence of aniridia was useful in the localization of a Wilms tumor gene (*WT1*) to chromosome 11p13 [reviewed in Reference 7]. In 1990, based on circumstantial evidence and theoretical grounds, it became evident that the *p53* tumor suppressor gene might be a viable candidate.

III. *p53*

In the early 1970s, Knudson compared the frequencies of familial cancers and their sporadic counterparts, using childhood retinoblastoma and Wilms tumor as theoretical models.[8] With statistical analysis, he suggested that the familial forms of these, and perhaps other, tumors could be explained by constitutional alterations of growth-limiting genes. Presumably, inactivation of the encoded proteins would facilitate cellular transformation.[9] Functional inactivation of these growth-limiting, or *tumor suppressor*, genes usually results either from mutations in both alleles, a mutation in one allele followed by a loss of or "reduction to homozygosity" in the second allele, or by functional or structural alteration of the protein product. Under this model, mutant tumor suppressor genes may be found either in germ cells or in somatic cells. In the former, they may arise *de novo* in the gamete or be transmitted from one generation to the next. Several tumor suppressor genes have now been isolated. Although the function of the protein encoded by each of these genes differs, virtually all share properties associated with suppression of cell growth and proliferation.[10] The *p53* tumor suppressor gene is associated with a variety of biological properties. A brief description of its structure and function are important to the discussion of its role in human cancer.

Alterations of the *p53* tumor suppressor gene and its encoded protein are the most frequently observed genetic events in human cancer.[11,12] The gene, located on human chromosome 17p13, encodes a 53-kDa nuclear phosphoprotein that appears to function as a negative regulator of cell growth and proliferation. Analysis of the nucleotide sequence of its 393 amino acids demonstrates 5 evolutionarily conserved domains in vertebrates.[13] The extent of conservation in invertebrates is unclear. The conserved regions are thought to be essential for the normal activity of p53. The p53 protein is characterized by the presence of binding sites for DNA tumor virus antigens, binding sites for at least one intracellular protein thought to influence the ability of p53 to transactivate other growth-regulatory genes, a nuclear localization signal, a transactivation signaling domain, an oligomerization domain, and several phosphorylation sites [Figure 2]. Extensive reviews of p53 structure and function are found elsewhere.[12,14-17]

The fact that p53 is frequently mutated or lost in many human tumors suggests that its normal function is that of a "growth suppressor".[11] The p53 protein binds specific DNA sequences and appears to act as a transcription factor that regulates the expression of other growth regulatory genes. Introduction of wild-type (normal) p53 protein into a variety of transformed cell types

Structural Features of p53

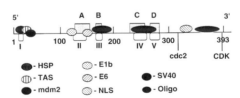

FIGURE 2. Structural features of the p53 tumor suppressor gene. The gene encodes a 53-kDa nuclear phosphoprotein. The 393 amino acids are spread over 11 exons. The transcription activation site (TAS), heat shock protein binding site (HSP), SV 40 large T antigen binding sites (SV40), nuclear localization signal (NLS), oligomerization domain (OLIGO), and phosphorylation sites (cdc2, a [315]Ser phosphorylated by p34[cdc2] kinase and CDK, a [392]Ser phosphorylated by casein kinase II) all identify potential functional regions. The five evolutionarily highly conserved domains (HCD I-V) correspond closely to the regions most frequently mutated in sporadic cancer (hot spot regions, HSR A-D). Sites of binding of the extracellular E1B-55-kDa protein of adenovirus type 5 (E1B), and the E6 gene product of human papilloma virus types 16 and 18 (E6) are also indicated, as is the position of the *MDM2* gene product binding site.

inhibits their growth [reviewed in Reference 12], most likely by blocking progression through the cell cycle at a checkpoint control site prior to G1/S. Also, p53 appears to play an important role in maintaining the fidelity of DNA repair, particularly in response to double-strand breaks induced either by ionizing radiation or by certain chemotherapeutic drugs.[16] Furthermore, recent work suggests that wild-type p53 could be involved in restricting precursor cell populations by mediating apoptosis (programmed cell death) in the absence of appropriate differentiation or proliferation signals.[16]

Several mechanisms can lead to inactivation of p53 function. Missense mutations, deletions, or nonsense mutations of the gene may alter the protein's conformation and prevent it from forming tetramers that bind specific DNA sequences to induce transcriptional activation of other growth-regulatory genes.[15] Inactivation of p53 may also occur through binding by other cellular proteins.[15] Some of the DNA tumor virus gene products, including SV40 T-antigen, the E1B 55-kDa protein of adenovirus type 5, and the E6 gene product of human papilloma virus types 16 and 18, encode proteins that bind to p53 [Figure 2]. In cells that co-express one of these viral oncoproteins along with p53, expression of p53-inducible reporter genes cannot be activated.[15] Disruption of normal p53 function may also be altered by alteration of *MDM2*, a cellular gene whose product has been shown to bind p53.[14] *MDM2* is amplified in a significant fraction of human sarcomas and, to a lesser extent, other tumors. The consequent overexpression of MDM2 probably interferes with p53 activity. In fact, recent evidence suggests that following radiation damage in a human fibroblast cell line, MDM2 mRNA levels increase, bind to wild-type p53, and terminate the transcriptional response to DNA damage mediated by wild-type p53.[18] MDM2 expression may therefore be part of a negative regulatory system designed to terminate the cell response to DNA damage.[18]

Although the precise function(s) of p53 are complex, a model has been proposed to account for many of these observations.[19] However, p53 is perhaps not required for normal cell division to occur. The levels of p53 normally rise in response to DNA damage, and the cell is arrested prior to the G1/S transition; the cell then undergoes either genomic repair or apoptosis. In those cells in which the p53 pathway is inactivated, G1 arrest does not occur and damaged DNA is replicated. As the cell undergoes mitosis, the presence of the damaged DNA may result in either mutation, aneuploidy, mitotic failure, and cell death. The surviving malignant clones may ultimately lead to cancer formation although numerous other genetic events are required to complete this process.[19]

IV. GERMLINE p53 MUTATIONS

A. THE LI-FRAUMENI SYNDROME

Mutations of the *p53* gene and alterations of the p53 protein have been associated with some fraction of virtually every sporadically occurring malignancy,[11,12] including all the cancer types found in LFS families.[4] Based on the hypothesis that the multi-site tumor phenotype seen in LFS might be accounted for by the same genetic mechanism involved in the development of tumors resulting from inactivations of *p53*, and supported by observations of multiple tumors in a *p53*-transgenic mouse model,[20] five LFS families were studied to determine whether *p53* played a role in the occurrence of cancer in the affected family members. By direct DNA sequencing, basepair mutations were identified in the germline of one or more affected members in each of the five families studied.[21] These were all missense mutations and were found in a short stretch within exon 7 — a highly conserved region of the protein. The remaining wild-type allele had been lost in the tumors from affected individuals.[21] Linkage analysis of one of these families, using a highly polymorphic DNA marker telomeric to *p53* on chromosome 17p (YNZ22.1), confirmed cosegregation of the abnormal *p53* allele with the polymorphism.[21] Gene carriers were identified among unaffected relatives, suggesting that they might be at risk of developing cancer at a later date. Shortly thereafter, a sixth LFS family was reported with a constitutional mutation in exon 7.[22] In this family, one affected member was not a carrier of the mutant gene, and might represent a sporadic case of cancer.

Several other families that fit our definition of LFS have since been studied and families with other germline *p53* mutations have been reported. One study of eight families from the Manchester childhood tumor registry suggested that mutations of the *p53* gene would not be found in all classic LFS families.[5] Only two of these eight families were found to carry germline mutations in exon 7. Further analyses of other exons did not identify mutations within exons 5 to 8 in several families. It is now believed that some classic LFS families do not have detectable germline mutations of the *p53* gene. In a recent analysis, 7 of 12 families conforming to a restricted definition of LFS harbored germline *p53* mutations. Although six of these were point mutations, one mutation in exon 4 was an unusual deletion/insertion alteration.[5] Only one of nine families with features less diagnostic of LFS harbored a germline *p53* mutation. The presence of childhood rhabdomyosarcoma, and to a slightly lesser extent adrenocortical carcinoma, was closely associated with the presence of germline *p53* mutations. These observations suggest that either of these tumors, in the context of a cancer family, would be associated with a particularly high risk of carrying a germline *p53* mutation.[5] Similar frequencies of germline p53 mutations in classic LFS families have been recently reported.[22a] There is at least one report of a typical LFS kindred in which overexpression of wild-type *p53* was observed in the absence of a *p53* gene mutation. This family suggests that the biologically or biochemically altered protein led to a similar phenotype, perhaps by one of the mechanisms described above.[23] Other reasons may also account for the lack of 100% concordance of germline *p53* mutations with the "classical" LFS phenotype. For example, alterations in other genes that are included in the development of cancers at multiple sites may give rise to a phenotype that resembles LFS. Defects in the promoter region of *p53* or in other genes that are involved in the *p53* growth-regulatory pathway may also yield the LFS phenotype. The presence of modifier genes may influence the phenotype that evolves from a specific gene mutation. With standard gene analysis, these abnormalities will not be detected. As the clinical definition of the syndrome is further refined, the association with *p53* mutations may become more apparent.

B. NON-LI-FRAUMENI SYNDROME

Recent improvements in DNA screening techniques[24] have made it possible to analyze large patient populations for the presence of constitutional abnormalities of the *p53* gene. These methods have led to the identification of certain "high-risk" patients and families who frequently carry germline *p53* mutations.

Germline *p53* mutations may be inherited from a carrier parent who has no clinical evidence of cancer at the time that the child is diagnosed with cancer. Presumably, acquisition of genetic events within the cell that ultimately gives rise to the malignant clone differs between parent and child and depends on many factors. The apparent phenotypic heterogeneity of LFS families has resulted in studies of non-LFS cancer-prone families, in order to characterize the heterogeneity of the *p53* carrier state.

Affected members in LFS kindreds often develop multiple primary neoplasms. One multicenter study demonstrated germline mutations of the *p53* tumor suppressor gene in four of 59 patients (6.8%) with second cancers, but who did not have family histories compatible with LFS at the time of their primary diagnosis.[25] One patient carried a heterozygous missense mutation at codon 248 in exon 7 that was identical to mutations previously described in LFS.[25] Mutations in codons 273 and 282 (a highly conserved region of exon 8 where *p53* mutations occur frequently in sporadic tumors) were identified in two patients. These mutations had not been previously reported in the germline. The fourth change involved a germline mutation in exon 9, affecting an amino acid residue that is conserved among mammals, but not lower vertebrates.[13] In addition to implicating codons outside the classically defined conserved regions of the *p53* gene, this study also demonstrated the occurrence of germline *p53* mutations in patients with cancers not commonly found in LFS, including non-Hodgkin's lymphoma, neuroblastoma, and colorectal and gastric carcinoma.

An extensive analysis of 196 patients (adults and children) with malignant sarcomas was reported together with the above study[26] — 8 patients (4%) harbored germline *p53* mutations; 5 of the 8 mutations were identified in patients from families with a high incidence of cancer. Both missense and nonsense germline mutations were found in this series. The latter all presumably yielded a truncated *p53* protein, although functional analysis of the *p53* product was not performed. This study also confirmed the observation of neutral polymorphisms within the *p53* sequence. One of these, at codon 213 in exon 6 (a nonconserved region), has been frequently identified in sporadic tumors.[13,26] It is important to be aware of the presence of such polymorphisms, especially if genetic counseling is performed. Without determining whether they are functionally significant, it is not possible to confirm their role in the causation of disease. This study also highlighted the variability of LFS. One family had an excess of gastric carcinomas, a tumor that had not been included in the operative definition of the syndrome. However, this family is from Japan, a country with a significantly higher incidence of gastric carcinoma than North American or European populations. It is possible, perhaps probable, that the background genetic make-up of the host may determine to a certain degree the cancer generated by the presence of a germline *p53* mutation. Environmental factors may also influence the type of tumors that arise in patients who carry *p53* germline mutations.

The LFS phenotype is most consistently characterized by the occurrence of sarcomas and multiple primary cancers in affected family members. Early onset breast cancers are also frequently encountered. Although acquired alterations of the *p53* gene or its encoded protein are frequently identified in the tissue of sporadic breast cancers, the frequency of germline *p53* mutations in breast cancer patients outside families with classical LFS is not known. A compilation of four studies of breast cancer patients ascertained by various criteria suggests that the frequency of germline *p53* mutations is less than 2%.[27-30] These findings suggest that germline *p53* mutations may occur rarely in early onset breast cancer outside of LFS. It is very likely that other genetic events are responsible for the genesis of this familial cancer clustering, and linkage studies have identified other breast cancer-predisposing loci.

Surveys of patients ascertained solely by the presence of a neoplasm that is a component tumor of LFS has yielded interesting observations. Adrenocortical carcinoma (ADCC) is a rare pediatric tumor, annually affecting only 3 per million children under the age of 16 years. However, in LFS kindreds, it is not uncommon to encounter at least one affected individual with ADCC.[4,5] Analysis of five patients with ADCC demonstrated inherited germline *p53* mutations in three.[31] Each of the families had pedigrees that were consistent with LFS. It has recently been reported that 50% of children with sporadic ADCC carry p53 mutations.[31a] A screen of primary lymphoblasts from 25 pediatric patients with acute lymphoblastic leukemia identified *p53* mutations in four, one of whom was shown to harbor the mutation (in exon 8) in the remission marrow, suggesting its germline origin.[32] The proband's pedigree was consistent with LFS. Analysis of primary lymphoblasts in affected members of ten familial leukemia pedigrees identified two families in whom nonhereditary *p53* alterations were present.[33] These studies suggest that although leukemia represents a common component tumor of LFS, germline *p53* mutation in leukemia patients is a rare event. Rhabdomyosarcoma (RMS), is the most frequently cited pediatric LFS tumor. In a survey of childhood RMS patients, 3/33 harbored germline p53 mutations in the absence of a family history of cancer. Interestingly, these mutations tended to occur in children with earlier onset disease.[33a] The occurrence of multiple primary tumors in affected LFS patients suggests that germline *p53* mutations could be found in nonfamilial patients with multiple primaries. A study of four patients with multifocal osteosarcoma and no family history of cancer demonstrated one apparently *de novo* germline *p53* mutation.[34] This observation suggested that other patients who present with multiple, nonfamilial cancers might also carry germline *p53* mutations.[34] The frequency of germline *p53* mutations in patients with gliomas with either multifocal disease, an additional primary malignancy, or a family history of cancer has been reported.[35] Of 51 glioma patients analyzed, 9 harbored germline *p53* mutations. In six of these, the patient had a multifocal tumor while the other three had unifocal disease with either a second malignancy or a family history that was consistent with LFS. The functional significance of some of the mutations described in this study was not confirmed. Osteosarcoma is frequently observed to occur in LFS. One multicenter study elected to determine the frequency of germline p53 mutations in a large series of pediatric osteosarcoma patients.[36] Of 235 patients analyzed, 7 (3.0%) were shown to carry heterozygous *p53* mutations. Four of these mutations were identified in children who did not have first-degree relatives with cancer. Taken together, these studies demonstrate that patients with germline *p53* mutations cannot be identified solely through a review of the family's cancer history [Figure 1 — right panel]. The method whereby the proband was ascertained will influence the frequency of carriers in the study population.

Although most reported germline *p53* mutations are missense, occasional nonsense mutations (base-pair deletions or insertions) have also been described.[5,13,37,38] Recently, splice mutations have also been found in the germline that are thought to disrupt the transcribed gene.[37,38a] Germline *p53* mutations are rarely distinct from somatic mutations. Furthermore, there has been no identifiable site-specific or tumor-limited expression of mutant *p53* alleles in the germline. Presumably, differences in genetic background between families account for variances in the LFS phenotype and the constellation of observed tumors.

As the pathobiologic characteristics of p53 are elucidated, it is important to establish the functional significance of germline *p53* mutations and the structural features of the corresponding mutant p53 proteins. In addition, the functional significance of a specific germline mutation must be carefully determined before one associates it with the development of cancer. The functional significance of heterozygous germline mutations in members of LFS families has been examined in several different systems[39-41] and it is apparent that certain germline p53 mutations might change the amino acid sequence in a conserved domain yet not be associated with inhibition of growth suppression or an increased cancer risk.

V. MOUSE MODELS OF THE p53 / LI-FRAUMENI SYNDROME

Transgenic mice that carry deregulated cancer-associated genes have proven to be valuable biologic models with which to study the molecular mechanisms that lead to cancer development. One attempt to determine whether p53 played a causative role in neoplasia and whether differences existed in cell type susceptibility was based on the use of transgenic mice that overexpress the mutant p53 protein.[20] The mice that were generated carried mutated *p53* genomic fragments under the control of their own promoters.[20] They also carried endogenous wild-type murine *p53* and therefore resembled the human Li-Fraumeni syndrome/*p53* genotype. The mutant transgene was expressed in a wide variety of tissues, including thymus, spleen, lymph nodes, and ovaries. Although neoplasms developed in 20% of the mice, intrinsic tissue-specific differences were suggested by the weak correlation between the degree of *p53* expression in certain tissues and the susceptibility to malignant transformation. In fact, the tumors were primarily osteosarcomas, lymphomas, and adenocarcinomas of the lung. This work contributed to the basis of the hypothesis that the distribution of neoplasms that occur in LFS might result from the transmission of a mutant *p53* gene.

Mouse *p53* has been implicated in cell-cycle control and might be important in normal embryonic development.[42] Homologous recombination in mouse embryonic stem cells was used to derive a null allele of the *p53* gene.[42] The mutated *p53* allele was established in the germline of chimeric mice with a mixed inbred genetic background (75% C57BL/6 and 25% 129/Sv). It was observed that mice homozygous for the mutated gene were viable and were apparently normal at birth. They were, however, susceptible to the spontaneous development of tumors before 6 months of age, predominantly lymphomas and hemangiosarcomas. Interestingly, multiple primary neoplasms of different cell types of origin were noted in 9 of the 26 tumor-bearing homozygote mice. The effect of genetic background on tumorigenesis in *p53*-deficient mice has been studied by inserting the same *p53* null allele as above into 129/Sv mice.[43] The most frequently observed tumor in these *p53*-deficient mice was again malignant lymphoma, but the spectrum of tumors differed from the mixed genotypic mice in that malignant teratocarcinomas were more common and hemangiosarcomas were less common. A third line of *p53* null mice (129/O1a) carrying a large deletion within *p53*, encompassing exons 2 through 6, demonstrates yet another spectrum of pathology. Crosses of the *p53*-transgenic mice with *p53*-deficient animals yields yet another distinct phenotype with a tendency to development of adenocarcinoma of the lung.[44a] These studies indicate that loss or alterations of p53 may accelerate tumor predisposition, and that the genetic background may play an important role in mediating the rate and spectrum of tumor development.

These studies have also demonstrated that p53-deficient mice are more sensitive to the effects of certain carcinogens. Exposure to liver-specific chemical carcinogens significantly decreases the survival of heterozygous, as compared to wild-type control mice.[44] Similar findings have been reported in a mouse skin carcinogenesis model in which heterozygous mice were treated with the initiator DMBA.[45] Although the mice developed a similar number of skin papillomas as their wild-type counterparts, a threefold increase in progression

TABLE 2
Incidence of Spontaneous Tumours in Selected p53-null and p53-transgenic Mice (%) Compared with Human LFS Counterpart

	Human LFS (variable genotype)	C57BL/6 × 129/Sv p53-/-	129/Sv p53-/-	CD-1 p53+/TG	129/O1a p53-/-	129/O1a p53+/-	C57BL/6 × 129/Sv × CD-1 p53+/-(Tg)
Lymphoma	-	65	75	36	82	35	40
Teratocarcinoma	-	35	9	2	-	-	-
Hemangiosarcoma	-	8	23	-	-	-	11
Osteosarcoma	6	8	5	36	-	18	9
Undiff. Sarcoma	2	-	7	-	-	-	3
Meningioma	-	4	-	-	-	-	-
Mammary adenoca.	26	4	2	-	-	-	3
Rhabdomyosarcoma	2	4	-	8	-	-	3
Leiomyosarcoma	10	4	-	-	-	-	3
Sarcoma (undefined)	-	-	-	-	23	35	-
Medulloblastoma	-	-	2	-	-	-	-
Schwanomma	-	-	2	-	-	-	-
Glioblastoma	1	-	2	-	-	-	-
Lung adenoca.	8	-	-	56	-	2	20
Skin carcinoma	-	-	-	8	-	-	3
Neuroblastoma	-	-	-	2	-	-	-
Astrocytoma	12	-	-	-	-	-	-
Melanoma	1	-	-	-	-	-	-
Prostate carcinoma	3	-	-	-	-	-	-
Pancreas carcinoma	3	-	-	-	-	-	-
Adrenocortical Ca.	2	-	-	-	-	-	-
Pituitary carcinoma	-	-	-	-	1	7	-
Pineoblastoma	-	-	-	-	-	-	-
Other	19	-	-	-	1	9	6

Note: Not all mouse models are represented due to incomplete phenotype data. The spectrum of tumors is apparently related both to modifier gene as well as p53 genotype factors. Adapted from References 20, 42, 44, and 44a.

to carcinomas was observed. It has yet to be determined whether equivalent observations will be observed in other carcinogen-induced tumors.

Similarities exist between the *p53* transgenic mouse models and LFS families. In both instances, a p53-related pathway of transformation leads to the development of a wide array of tumors. The inheritance of one wild-type *p53* gene and one mutant gene observed in LFS families is analogous to the heterozygote mice who develop spontaneous tumors at a slow rate. It remains to be seen whether heterozygous mice with a single null allele develop tumors through molecular pathways similar to LFS patients. Those mutations in the human germline that yield a truncated (and presumably inactive) p53 protein may represent the inherited cancer syndrome for which the p53-deficient mice are a genetically accurate animal model.[43]

VI. PREDICTIVE TESTING IN THE LI-FRAUMENI SYNDROME

The identification of germline mutations of the *p53* tumor suppressor gene in rare cancer-prone families has introduced several complex issues. These include such practical problems as clarification of the definition of LFS, determination of the functional significance of somatic and germline mutations in cancer patients generally, and the development of practical and accurate laboratory techniques to confirm mutations. Ethical questions of screening and predictive testing address the selection of patients to be tested, the development of pilot programs in research and service settings, the means of transmission of results to test subjects, their affected and unaffected relatives and interested third parties, and the potential roles for preventive and therapeutic interventions based on test results. Many of these issues are discussed elsewhere in this volume as they apply to familial cancer in general.

For several reasons, p53 testing should not at present be offered to the general population. Even within the general cancer population the carrier rate is low,[4,6] the frequency of germline *p53* mutations likely being less than 1% of all cancers. The sensitivity and specificity of screening methods to identify mutations are not known and both false-positive and false-negative results may occur. Even the sequence-confirmed presence of a base-pair alteration must itself be interpreted carefully in that it should in some way lead to inactivation of normal p53 function.

The clinical implications of germline *p53* mutations are not accurately known. For these reasons, it is generally accepted that screening of unaffected individuals be restricted to blood relatives of LFS families or cancer cases with documented germline *p53* mutations.[44] Effective ways must be developed to provide informed consent to those being screened about the potential beneficial and harmful psychologic and social sequelae of participation in these screening programs. The development of multidisciplinary screening programs should address aspects of cost, informed consent — particularly where it affects children — socioeconomic impact on the individual tested, and consistency in providing results and counseling.[46]

Generally, the component malignancies of LFS are difficult to cure, and only partly amenable to preclinical screening. Furthermore, it is not clear to what extent early identification reduces mortality. Chemoprevention may be of some value in certain cancers, but is not of universal benefit. These factors must be accounted for in the approach to counseling of at-risk patients.

The possibility of reducing the marked loss of human potential that results from the death of a child or young adult makes studies of the genetics of hereditary cancer syndromes particularly worthwhile. The development of accurate testing techniques, a better understanding of the biologic effect of germline mutations, and the evaluation of animal models will continue to be important. One hopes that these studies will lead through screening to the early detection and successful treatment of cancer.

ACKNOWLEDGMENTS

The author is a Scholar of the Medical Research Council of Canada and is supported by grants from the Medical Research Council of Canada and the National Cancer Institute of Canada.

REFERENCES

1. **Li, F. P. and Fraumeni, J. F., Jr.,** Soft-tissue sarcomas, breast cancer, and other neo-plasms: a familial syndrome? *Ann. Intern. Med.*, 71, 747, 1969.
2. **Li, F. P. and Fraumeni, J. F., Jr.,** Rhabdomyosarcoma in children: epidemiologic study and identification of a familial cancer syndrome. *J. Natl. Cancer Inst.*, 43, 1365, 1969.
3. **Li, F. P., Fraumeni, J. F. Jr., Mulvihill, J. J., Blattner, W. A., Dreyfus, M. G., Tucker, M. A., and Miller, R. W.,** A cancer family syndrome in twenty-four kindreds. *Cancer Res.*, 48, 5358, 1988.
4. **Garber, J. E., Goldstein, A. M., Kantor, A. F., Dreyfus, M. G., Fraumeni, J. F., Jr., and Li, F. P.,** Follow-up study of twenty-four families with Li-Fraumeni syndrome. *Cancer Res.*, 51, 6094, 1991.
5. **Birch, J. M., Hartley, A. L., Tricker, K. J., Prosser, J., Condie, A., Kelsey, A. M., Harris, M., Morris-Jones, P. H., Binchy, A., Crowther, D., Craft, A. W., Eden, O. B., Evans, G. R., Thompson, E., Mann, J. R., Martin, J., Mitchell, E. L. D., and Santibañez-Koref, M. F.,** Prevalence and diversity of constitutional mutations in the p53 gene among 21 Li-Fraumeni families. *Cancer Res.*, 54, 1298, 1994.
6. **Williams, W. R. and Strong, L.C .,** Genetic epidemiology of soft tissue sarcomas in children. In Muller, H. R. and Weber, W. (Eds.): *Familial Cancer. First International Research Conference,* S. Karger, Basel, 1985, 151.
7. **Pelletier, J.,** Molecular genetics of Wilms' tumor: insights into normal and abnormal renal development. *Can. J. Oncol.,* 4, 262, 1994.
8. **Knudson, A. G.,** Mutation and cancer: statistical study of retinoblastoma. *Proc. Natl. Acad. Sci. U.S.A.,* 68, 820, 1971.
9. **Comings, D. E.,** A general theory of carcinogenesis. *Proc. Natl. Acad. Sci. U.S.A.,* 70, 3324, 1973.
10. **Levine, A. J.,** *Tumor Suppressor Genes, The Cell Cycle and Cancer.* Vol 12. Cold Spring Harbor Laboratory Press, Cold Spring Harbor, NY, 1992, 1.
11. **Harris, C. C. and Hollstein, M.,** Clinical implications of the p53 tumor-suppressor gene. *N. Engl. J. Med.,* 329, 1318, 1993.
12. **Nigro, J. M., Baker, S. J., Preisinger, A. C., Jessup, J., Hotsetter, R., Cleary, K., Bigner, S., Davidson, N., Baylin, S., Devilee, P., and Vogelstein, B.,** Mutations in the p53 gene occur in diverse human tumor types. *Nature,* 342, 705, 1989.
13. **Caron de Fromentel, C. and Soussi, T.,** TP suppressor gene: a model for investigating human mutagenesis. *Genes Chrom. Cancer,* 4, 1, 1992.
14. **Levine, A. J.,** *N. Engl. J. Med.,* 326, 1350, 1992.

15. **Vogelstein, B. and Kinzler, K. W.,** p53 Function and dysfunction. *Cell*, 70, 523, 1992.

16. **Donehower, L. A. and Bradley, A.,** The tumor suppressor p53. *Biochem. Biophys. Acta*, 1155, 181, 1993.

17. **Harris, C. C.,** *Science*, 262, 1980, 1993.

18. **Price, B. D. and Park, S. J.,** DNA damage increases the levels of MDM2 messenger RNA in wtp53 human cells. *Cancer Res.*, 54, 896, 1994.

19. **Lane, D. P.,** p53, Guardian of the genome. *Nature*, 358, 15, 1992.

20. **Lavigueur, A., Maltby, V., Mock, D., Rossant, J., Pawson, T., and Bernstein, A.,** High incidence of lung, bone, and lymphoid tumors in transgenic mice overexpressing mutant alleles of the p53 oncogene. *Mol. Cell Biol.*, 9, 3982, 1989.

21. **Malkin, D., Li, F. P., Strong, L. C., Fraumeni, J. F., Jr., Nelson, C. E., Kim, D. H., Kassel, J., Gryka, M. A., Bischoff, F. Z., Tainsky, M. A., and Friend, S. H.,** Germline p53 mutations in a familial syndrome of breast cancer, sarcomas, and other neoplasms. *Science*, 250, 1233, 1990.

22. **Srivastava, S., Zou, Z. Q., Pirollo, K., Blattner, W., and Chang, E. H.,** Germ line transmission of a mutated p53 gene in a cancer-prone family with Li-Fraumeni syndrome. *Nature*, 348, 747, 1990.

22a. **Frebourg, T., Barbier, N., Yan, Y., Garber, J. E., Dreyfus, M., Fraumeni, J., Jr., Li, F. P., and Friend, S. H.,** Germ-line p53 mutations in 15 families with Li-Fraumeni syndrome. *Am. J. Hum. Genet.*, 56, 608, 1995.

23. **Barnes, D. M., Hanby, A. M., Gillett, C. E., Mohammed, S., Hodgson, S., Bobrow, L. G., Leigh, I. M., Purkis, T., MacGeoch, C., Spurr, N. K., Bartek, J., Vojtesek, B., Picksley, S. M., and Lane, D. P.,** Abnormal expression of wild-type p53 protein in normal cells of a cancer family patient. *Lancet*, 2, 340, 259, 1992.

24. **Prosser, J.,** Detecting single-base mutations. *Trends Biotechnol.*, 11, 238, 1993.

25. **Malkin, D., Jolly, K. W., Barbier, N., Look, A. T., Friend, S. H., Gebhardt, M C., Andersen, T. I., Borresen, A.-L., Li, F. P., Garber, J., and Strong, L. C.,** Germline mutations of the p53 tumor suppressor gene in children and young adults with second malignant neoplasms. *N. Engl. J. Med.*, 326, 1309, 1992.

26. **Toguchida, J., Yamaguchi, T., Dayton, S. H., Beauchamp, R. L., Herrera, G. E., Ishizaki, K., Yamamuro, T., Meyers, P. A., Little, J. B., Sasaki, M. S., Weichselbaum, R. R., and Yandell, D. W.,** Prevalence and spectrum of germline mutations of the p53 gene among patients with sarcoma. *N. Engl. J. Med.*, 326, 1301, 1992.

27. **Prosser, J., Elder, P. A., Condie, A., MacFayden, I., Steel, C. M., and Evans, H. J.,** Mutations in p53 do not account for heritable breast cancer: a study in five affected families. *Br. J. Cancer*, 63, 181, 1991.

28. **Warren, W., Eeles, R. A., Ponder, B. A. J., Easton, D. F., Averill, D., Ponder, M. A., Anderson, K., Evans, A. M., DeMars, R., Love, R., Dundas, S., Stratton, M. R., Trowbridge, P., Copper, C. S., and Peto, J.,** No evidence for germline mutations in exons 5-9 of the p53 gene in 25 breast cancer families. *Oncogene*, 7, 1043, 1992.

29. **Børresen A.-L., Andersen, T. I., Garber, J., Barbier, N., Thorlacius, S., Eyfjord, J., Ottestad, L., Smith-Sorrensen, B., Hovig, E., Malkin, D., and Friend, S. H.,** Screening for germ line TP 53 mutations in breast cancer patients. *Cancer Res.*, 52, 3234, 1992.

30. **Sidransky, D., Tokino, T., Helzlsouer, K., Zehnbauer, B., Rausch, G., Shelton, B., Prestigiacomo, L., Vogelstein, B., and Davidson, N.,** Inherited p53 gene mutations in breast cancer. *Cancer Res.*, 52, 2984, 1992.

31. **Sameshima, Y., Tsunematsu, Y., and Watanabe, S.,** Detection of novel germline p53 mutations in diverse cancer-prone families identified by selecting patients with childhood adrenocortical carcinoma. *J. Natl. Cancer Inst.*, 84, 703, 1992.

31a. **Wagner, J., Portwine, C., Rabin, K., Leclerc, J-M., Narod, S. A., and Malkin, D.,** High frequency of germline p53 mutations in childhood adrenocortical cancer. *J. Natl. Cancer Inst.* 86, 1707, 1994.

32. **Felix, C. A., Nau, M. M., Takahashi, T., Mitsudomi, T., Chiba, I., Poplack, D. G., Reaman, G. H., Cole, D. E., Letterio, J. J., Whang-Peng, J., Knutsen, T., and Minna, J. D.,** Hereditary and acquired p53 gene mutations in childhood acute lymphoblastic leukemia. *J. Clin. Invest.,* 89, 640, 1992.

33. **Felix, C. A., D'Amico, D., Mitsudomi, T., Nau, M.M., Li, F. P., Fraumeni, J. F., Jr., Cole, D. E., McCalla, J., Reaman, G. H., Whang-Peng, J., Knutsen, T., Minna, J. D., and Poplack, D. G.,** Absence of hereditary p53 mutations in 10 familial leukemia pedigrees. *J. Clin. Invest.,* 90, 653, 1992.

33a. **Diller, L., Sexsmith, E., Gottlieb, A., Li, F. P., and Malkin, D.,** Germline p53 mutations are frequently detected in young children with rhabdomyosarcoma. *J. Clin. Invest.,* 95, 1606, 1995.

34. **Iavarone, A., Matthay, K. K., Steinkirchner, T. M., and Israel, M. A.,** Germline and somatic p53 gene mutations in multifocal osteogenic sarcoma. *Proc. Natl. Acad. Sci. U.S.A.,* 89, 4207, 1992.

35. **Kyritsis, A. P., Bondy, M. L., Xiao, M., Berman, E. L., Cunningham, J. E., Lee, P. S., Levin, V. A., and Saya, H.,** Germline mutations in subsets of glioma patients. *J. Natl. Cancer Inst.,* 86, 344, 1994.

36. **McIntyre, J. F., Smith-Sorensen, B., Friend, S. H., Kassel, J., Borresen, A.-L., Yan, Y.-X., Russo, C., Sato, J., Barbier, N., Miser, J., Malkin, D., and Gebhardt, M. C.,** Germline mutations of the p53 tumor suppressor gene in children with osteosarcoma. *J. Clin. Oncol.,* 12, 925, 1994.

37. **Felix, C. A., Strauss, E. A., D'Amico, D., Tsokos, M., Winter, S., Mitsudomi, T., Nau, M. M., Brown, D. L., Leahey, A. M., Horowitz, M. E., Poplack, D. G., Costin, D., and Minna, J. D.,** A novel germline p53 splicing mutation in a pediatric patient with a second malignant neoplasm. *Oncogene,* 8, 1203, 1993.

38. **Jolly, K. W., Malkin, D., Douglass, E. C., Brown, T. F., Sinclair, A. E., and Look, A. T.,** Splice-site mutation of the p53 gene in a family with hereditary breast-ovarian cancer. *Oncogene,* 9, 97, 1994.

38a. **Warneford, S. G., Witton, L. J., Townsend, M. L., Rowe, P. B., Reddel, R. R., Dalla-Pozza, L., and Symonds, G.,** Germ-line splicing mutation of the p53 gene in a cancer-prone family. *Cell Growth Different.,* 3, 839, 1992.

39. **Srivastava, S., Tong, Y.A., Devadas, K., Zou, Z.-Q., Sykes, V. W., Chen, Y., Blattner, W. A., Pirollo, K., and Chang, E. H.,** Detection of both mutant and wild-type p53 protein in normal skin fibroblasts and demonstration of a shared "second-hit" on p53 in diverse tumors from a cancer-prone family with Li-Fraumeni syndrome. *Oncogene,* 7, 987, 1992.

40. **Frebourg, T., Barbier, N., Kassel, J., Ng, Y. S., Romero, P., and Friend, S. H.,** A functional screen for germ line p53 mutations based on transcriptional activation. *Cancer Res.,* 52, 6976, 1992.

41. **Ishioka, C., Frebourg, T., Yan, Y.-X., Vidal, M., Friend, S. H., Schmidt, S., and Iggo, R.,** Screening patients for heterozygous p53 mutations using a functional assay in yeast. *Nat. Genet.,* 5, 124, 1993.

42. **Donehower, L. A., Harvey, M., Slagle, B.L., McArthur, M. J., Montgomery, C. A., Jr., Butel, J., and Bradley, A.,** Mice deficient for p53 are developmentally normal but susceptible to spontaneous tumors. *Nature,* 356, 215, 1992.

43. **Harvey, M., McArthur, M. J., Montgomery, C. A., Jr., Butel, J. S., Bradley, A., and Donehower, L. A.,** Genetic background alters the spectrum of tumors that develop in p53-deficient mice. *FASEB J.,* 7, 938, 1993.

44. **Harvey, M., McArthur, M. J., Montgomery, C. A., Jr., Butel, J. S., Bradley, A., and Donehower, L. A.,** Spontaneous and carcinogen-induced tumorigenesis in p53-deficient mice. *Nat. Genet.,* 5, 225, 1993.

44a. **Harvey, M., Vogel, H., Morris, D., Bradley, A., Bernstein, A., and Donehower, L. A.,** A mutant p53 transgene accelerates tumour development in heterozygous but not nullizygous p53-deficient mice. *Nature Genet.*, 9, 305, 1995.

45. **Kemp, C. J., Donehower, L. A., Bradley, A., and Balmain, A.,** Reduction of p53 gene dosage does not increase initiation or promotion but enhances malignant progression of chemically induced skin tumors. *Cell*, 74, 813, 1993.

46. **Li, F. P., Garber, J. E., Friend, S. H., Strong, L. C., Patinaude, A. F., Juengst, E. T., Reilly, P. R., Correa, P., and Fraumeni, J. F., Jr.,** Recommendations on predictive testing for germline p53 mutations among cancer-prone individuals. *J. Natl. Cancer Inst.*, 84, 1156, 1992.

Chapter 6

CLINICAL DIAGNOSIS OF FAMILIAL CANCER

Walter Weber

CONTENTS

I. DEFINITION

There is *no consensus* on the definition of a cancer family. In industrialized countries about one in four inhabitants develops cancer. Therefore, most persons have one or more relatives with cancer, just by chance; 6% of cancer patients are reported to have three or more first-degree relatives with cancer.[1] About half of the cancer patients had no first-degree relatives with cancer, 30% had one, and 12% had two; 15% of patients with breast or colorectal cancer had one to three first-degree relatives with the same disease.[2]

Our *working definition* of familial cancer is two or more first-degree relatives (parent, sister, brother, or child) affected by cancer diagnosed by microscopic examination. Sporadic cancer, then, is defined as one cancer in first-degree relatives of a family.

II. TAKING A HISTORY

Medical interviewing is one of the most important activities of every doctor. Learning these skills is often left to chance, unfortunately. It is an important duty of medical schools to teach medical interviewing.[3]

Every person has a story that demonstrates the interaction among the biologic, psychologic, and social components of his or her life. The physician's task is to elicit and understand this story, for it provides an introduction to who

0-8493-4782-3/96/$0.00+$.50
© 1996 by CRC Press Inc.

the person is and why she or he is seeing the physician. It also provides clues to preventive, diagnostic, and therapeutic issues relevant to the patient's problem.[4] Taking a personal and family history is an important part of the medical interview.

Familial cancer aggregations are brought to the physician's attention by a patient or a healthy person with an affected near relative.

The personal history is the starting point of an interview by familial cancer professionals. For this purpose the medical history questionnaire for cancer etiology of the U.S. National Cancer Institute may be of use.[5] It focuses in its first part on identifying carcinogenic exposures. As a reference the Monographs of the International Agency for Research on Cancer (IARC) in Lyon, France is recommended.[6] The occupational and environmental history is important in this respect.[7,8] The personal history can also give clues for hereditary cancer predispositions (Table 1).

The family history is the main task of a familial cancer professional. It gives us basic information for all future measures. There are certain features suggestive of a hereditary cancer predisposition in a family (Table 2).

TABLE 1
Features Suggestive of a Hereditary Cancer Predisposition in a Cancer Patient

- Multiple primary tumors in the same organ
- Multiple primary tumors in different organs
- Bilateral primary tumors
- Multifocality
- Young age at tumor diagnosis
- At unusual site (s)
- Rare histology
- In the sex not usually affected
- Associated with genetic traits
- Associated with congenital defects
- Associated with a precursor lesion
- Associated with a rare disease

TABLE 2
Features Suggestive of a Hereditary Cancer Predisposition in a Family

- One first-degree relative with a tumor and with any of the features listed in Table 1
- Two or more first-degree relatives with tumors of the same localization
- Two or more first-degree relatives with tumor localizations belonging to known familial cancer syndromes
- Two or more first-degree relatives with rare tumors
- Three or more relatives in two generations with tumors of the same localization

Generally accepted *symbols* should be used for a pedigree in order to facilitate professional communication (Figures 1 and 2). Certain *rules* should be observed: every person of a family must be noted down. The sequence of births should be derivable, every stillbirth and abortion included. Every family member is given a unique number (generation: Roman digit, position within a generation: Arabian digit).

A list should be generated containing the following data for every family member: number in the pedigree, name, maiden name, first name; date and place of birth; affected by cancer — if yes: cancer localization, microscopy diagnosis, date of diagnosis; survival status, if dead: date and cause of death; diseases and peculiarities; addresses (own, treating physicians, hospitals, etc.).

Anamnestic data should be verified as far as possible by obtaining copies of medical and pathology reports and verified information should be registered, be it positive or negative. Usually, the interviewed patient (proband) agrees to mediate contacts with his relatives. Their physicians should also be informed and agree.

The family history approach is a low-technology procedure applicable all over the world. What it needs is interest, time, and patience. Information from one person can be completed and deepened by asking other family members. The sources of the information should also be noted.

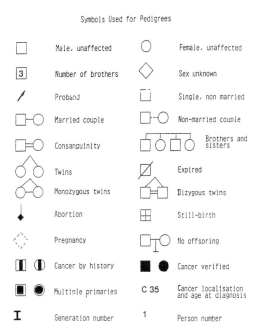

FIGURE 1.

PEDIGREE

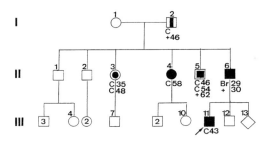

FIGURE 2.

The accuracy of a cancer patient's report of cancer among relatives is respectable. In one study the primary cancer site was correct in 83% of first-degree, 67% of second-degree, and 60% of third-degree relatives.[9]

A simple contribution *everybody* could make to his health is to *write down his own family history*. First, make a list of all first-degree relatives — parents, sisters, brothers, and children. Then list all serious illnesses they have had and their age at diagnosis. Include age and cause of death when appropriate. Ask close female relatives — mother, grandmother, and aunts about illnesses such as breast and reproductive cancers. The next time you visit your physician, take the list and discuss your health risks and what you can do to lessen them.

III. THE PHYSICAL EXAMINATION

Physical signs are objective and verifiable marks of disease. Their significance is enhanced when they confirm a change already suggested by the history. At times, the physical signs may be the only evidence of disease.

The physical examination should be performed methodically and thoroughly, with due regard for the patient's comfort and modesty. The examination must extend from head to toe in an objective search for abnormalities. The results should be recorded at the time they are elicited. Inaccuracies stem from distortions of the memory.

Skill in physical diagnosis is acquired with experience combined with a mind prepared to be alert to certain findings. Physical findings are subject to change. It is important, therefore, to repeat pertinent parts of the physical examination.

Preneoplastic and neoplastic syndromes can be recognized by physical examination, searching for dysmorphic features, congenital anomalies, or abnormal cutaneous manifestations, which are often unreported.[10]

Discoveries in medicine often come about from observations made at the bedside.[11] From the history and physical examination the alert practitioner can identify clues to risk factors for specific cancers.[12]

IV. FURTHER DIAGNOSTIC METHODS

For information on further diagnostic approaches and methods (e.g., imaging techniques) standard oncology textbooks should be consulted. Laboratory methods relevant in familial cancer are presented in this book. A definite oncologic diagnosis requires cytologic and/or histologic investigations.

V. PATHOLOGY

Familial tumors appear in many histologic forms just as do sporadic tumors. They both look the same under the microscope. The relative distribution of histologic subtypes may be different in familial cancer as opposed to sporadic cancer. In breast cancer, lobular histologic characteristics may be associated in some instances with an increased risk to relatives.[13] Mucinous carcinoma has been considered a feature of colorectal cancer in hereditary nonpolyposis colorectal cancer.[14] Medullary thyroid carcinoma is predominant in the inherited multiple endocrine neoplasia syndromes.[15] Pathology features are described elsewhere in this book.

REFERENCES

1. **Weber, W.,** The potential of the familial cancer registry for anticancer research and medical practice. *Anticancer Res.* 6: 701–704, 1986.
2. **Weber, W.,** Cancer control by family history, *Anticancer Res.,* 13: 1197–1202, 1993.
3. **Lipkin, M., Quill, T. E., and Napodano, R. J.,** The medical interview: a core curriculum for residences in internal medicine. *Ann. Intern. Med.* 100: 277–284, 1984.
4. **Smith, R. C. and Hoppe, R. B.,** The patient's story: integrating the patient- and physician-centered approaches to interviewing. *Ann. Intern. Med.* 115: 470–477, 1991.
5. **Appendix.** In: *Genetics of Human Cancer,* edited by J. J. Mulvihill, R. W. Miller, and J. F. Fraumeni, Jr., Raven Press, New York, pp 489–493, 1977.
6. IARC Monographs on the Evaluation of Carcinogenic Risks to Humans, World Health Organisation, Distribution and Sales, Geneva, Switzerland.

7. The Occupational and Environmental Health Committee of the American Lung Association of San Diego and Imperial Counties. Taking the occupational history. *Ann. Intern. Med.* 99: 641–651, 1983.

8. American College of Physicians. Occupational and environmental medicine: the internist's role. *Ann. Intern. Med.* 113: 974–982, 1990.

9. **Love, R. R., Evans, A. M., and Josten, D. M.,** The accuracy of patient reports of a family history of cancer. *J. Chronic Dis.* 38: 289–293, 1985.

10. **Fusaro, R. M.,** The environment and cancer-associated genodermatoses, in *Genetic Epidemiology of Cancer*, Lynch, H. T. and Hirayama T., Eds., CRC Press, Boca Raton, FL, 159–185, 1989.

11. **Miller, R. W.,** Rare events as clues to cancer etiology. *Cancer Res.* 48, 3544–3548, 1988.

12. **Miller, R. W.,** The discovery of human teratogens, carcinogens, and mutagens: lessons for the future, in *Chemical Mutagens*, Hollaender, A. and Serres, F. J., Eds., Plenum Press, New York, 101–126, 1978.

13. **Claus, E. B., Risch, N., Thompson, W. D., and Carter, D.,** Relationship between breast histopathology and family history of breast cancer. *Cancer* 71: 147–153, 1993.

14. **Lynch, H. T., Smyrk, T. C., Watson, P., Lanspa, S. J., Lynch, J. F., Lynch, P. M., Cavalivi, R. J., and Boland C. R.,** Genetics, natural history, tumor spectrum, and pathology of hereditary nonpolyposis colorectal cancer: an updated review. *Gastroenterology* 104: 1535–1549, 1993.

15. **Gardner, E., Papi, L., Easton, D. F., Cummings, T., Jackson, C. E., Kaplan, M., Love, D. R., Mole, S. E., Moore, J. K., Mulligan, L. M., Norum, R. A., Ponder, M. A., Reichlin, S., Stall, G., Telenius, H., Telenius-Berg, M., Tunnacliffe, A., and Ponder, B. A. J.,** Genetic linkage studies map the multiple endocrine neoplasia type 2 loci to a small interval on chromosome 10q11.2. *Hum. Mol. Genet.* 2: 241–246, 1993.

Chapter 7

LABORATORY DIAGNOSIS OF FAMILIAL CANCER

Rodney J. Scott

CONTENTS

I. INTRODUCTION

Laboratory procedures that have become available since the advent of molecular biology nowadays make possible the accurate identification of affected persons coming from families where there is an overrepresentation of disease compared to the general population. Prior to any laboratory investigation concerning familial cancer, an accurate medical diagnosis is required such that laboratory investigators can narrow the spectrum of choices that are taken to ensure an efficient and meaningful course in their investigations. The clinician and the laboratory investigator must work hand in hand to provide not only an accurate diagnosis of disease but also a reliable assessment of risk for any given family member. As our understanding of the biology of malignant

0-8493-4782-3/96/$0.00+$.50

disease increases, so does our power to accurately diagnose persons who have an increased risk of disease development.

II. IDENTIFICATION OF FAMILIES AND SAMPLE COLLECTION

The most readily studied familial diseases tend to be autosomal dominant, as it is usually apparent when persons have inherited a particular trait. Autosomal recessive disorders are more often diagnosed when a single patient is identified with a specific disease. Familial studies in this instance could be performed, but acquisition of affected persons may be difficult when rigorous testing is required. As a corollary to this, among families coming from cultures where consanguinity is most frequent, recessive diseases are very much more prevalent.

The first and by far the most important aspect of any laboratory diagnosis of familial cancer is an accurate anamnestic questioning of the proband to determine if, in fact, a person comes from a family that does have a predisposition to a particular disease. As cancer is a very common disease, the chances that two persons coming from the same family will develop the same illness are relatively high (approximately 1 in 1,000). It is estimated, for instance, that should a person develop colorectal cancer their relatives will also have an increased predisposition to develop it.[1] More precisely, the likelihood that two persons coming from the same family will develop cancer are relatively high (about 1 in 9). Should three persons from the same family suffer the same malignancy, the probability of this occurring by chance alone decreases significantly to about 1 in 250.[2] Therefore, should a patient say that his brother, mother, and aunt have all had the same cancer then it is likely that this family belongs to one of the cancer family syndromes. Families where there are more than three first-grade relatives affected with the same disease are extremely rare and represent very good evidence of a genetic predisposition. Unfortunately, in the situation where three or less first-degree persons or fewer are affected the evidence of a genetic predisposition is very much weaker; however, as these families are much more common their cumulative information could indicate a genetic predisposition.

An additional and important factor that needs to be remembered is the problem of penetrance. Penetrance of a particular trait may severely influence a decision as to whether there is a family history of disease. For many cases of familial cancer, this is not a problem. For instance, in the autosomal dominant disease of familial adenomatous polyposis (FAP), the likelihood someone will develop symptoms given that they have a genetic predisposition is virtually 100% by the age of 40,[3] whereas for breast cancer the lifetime risk is approximately 80% in carriers of BRCA1.[4] It must also be borne in mind with respect to breast cancer that it is primarily a disease of women, such that the disease may disappear in one generation but reappear in the next, as illustrated in Figure 1.

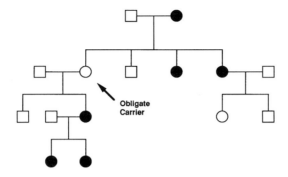

FIGURE 1. Pedigree of a family with breast cancer showing incomplete penetrance due to the disease not being expressed in the mother of the individual identified.

For a molecular genetic diagnosis to be made, several criteria need to be considered. At the time of diagnosis, a blood sample should be taken from the patient, usually 20 ml EDTA blood and 20 ml heparin blood. EDTA blood is required for immediate isolation of DNA, whereas lymphocytes are isolated from heparin blood and immortalized with Epstein-Barr virus such that a continuous source of DNA is available for analysis (this is especially important due to the nature of neoplastic disease). It is an absolute requirement to have at least two affected living persons (first-degree relatives) who preferably have been ascertained prior to medical intervention, and two unaffected first-degree relatives. All persons at risk of having inherited the predisposition should also be encouraged to provide a blood sample. Blood collection is preferred treatment as the patient may undergo therapy that can alter his/her genetic profile, leading to spurious results.

III. LABORATORY METHODS USED FOR DIAGNOSIS

Before a diagnosis of a familial cancer can be made, an approximation as to where a particular disease gene lies in the genome must be known. Until the gene locus is known, the only reliable diagnosis of a familial trait is by pedigree inspection.

Essentially, to date, two methods have been employed for the isolation of genes associated with inherited susceptibilities. These are functional cloning and positional cloning. The two methods differ in that the former is based on information that is already known, such as an enzyme defect or a failure in receptor ligand binding. Positional cloning, however, cannot make use of such functional differences and therefore relies on a slightly different approach. The genetic or physical location of the disease gene in the genome is required, with little if any knowledge of the gene's function.[5] Two recent examples of such an approach are the genes that have been identified that predispose to colorectal cancer and breast cancer development.

A. INDIRECT GENETIC ANALYSIS

Indirect genetic analysis implies that a susceptibility gene for a given disease exists although its exact whereabouts remains elusive. Before a susceptibility gene can be located within a specific manageable sequence of DNA that can then be more intensively evaluated, an approximation as to where it lies in the genome is required. Investigations had previously sought to identify gross phenotypic alterations with chromosomal changes that may have occurred in association with a specific disease. This method of detective work proved quite successful in the search for the gene predisposing to FAP. The gene locus in this instance was identified from a severely retarded patient who also had polyposis coli.[6] Since the development of polymerase chain reaction (PCR) technology and the identification of many markers on the human genome, new strategies have become available for the identification of genes predisposing to particular traits. A recent example of the combination of PCR technology and the information gained from the human genome project culminated in the identification of genes[7] that are responsible for hereditary nonpolyposis colorectal cancer (HNPCC). Other examples also exist, such as the *BRCA1* gene locus which is associated with familial breast cancer.[8]

Linkage analysis remains the major method by which risk assessment is determined and this involves both molecular genetic investigations and computer analysis using the linkage programs developed by Lathrop and coworkers.[9] Linkage analysis has become much easier and thanks, in part, are due to the results of the human genome project, which has helped identify repetitive sequences that can be used for this analysis. The analysis of simple repeated sequences are generally much more informative than restriction fragment length polymorphism analysis (RFLP), making linkage studies very much faster. Although RFLP analysis is slowly disappearing, it remains a useful tool in the diagnosis of some inherited disorders and is still employed in the search for candidate genes.

1. Restriction Fragment Length Polymorphism Analysis

Essentially, differences between DNA obtained from different family members can be treated as allelic variants either of a gene or close to a gene and used as genetic markers for gene mapping. Such differences can be visualized using the technique first described by Southern in 1975.[10] This technique relies on the presence of restriction endonuclease (RE) sites throughout the genome that are recognized by restriction enzymes which cut DNA at these sites (shown schematically in Figure 2). The resulting DNA fragments are of different lengths which can be size fractionated on agarose gel as depicted in Figure 3a. If the DNA sequence is the same from one allele to another no difference between the two can be discerned, implying that it is not polymorphic. More often, however, there are differences as to where RE sites occur in homologous

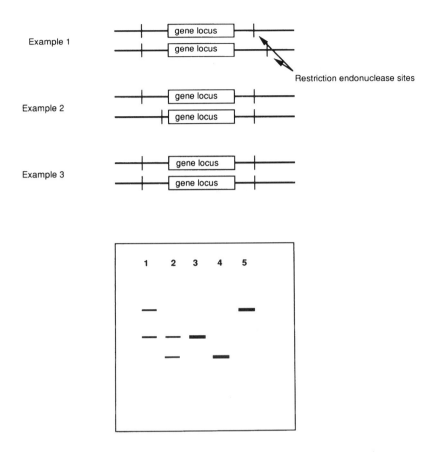

FIGURE 2. A diagrammatic representation of a Southern blot, indicating heterozygous alleles and homozygous alleles.

chromosomes and this results in fragments of DNA being unequal in length. The resulting difference in size can be used as a flag to establish if a particular length of DNA segregates with a disease. Visualization of such differences in the size of cut DNA is relatively straightforward. Briefly, the cut DNA is (after electrophoretic size fractionation) denatured, transferred to an inert membrane, and hybridized to a complementary piece of radioactively labeled (usually ^{32}P) DNA. Once hybridized, the membrane is placed in contact with autoradiographic film and exposed for two to three days. An example is shown in Figure 3b. The results of such investigations are referred to as restriction fragment length polymorphisms (RFLPs). RFLPs have no function and therefore do not interfere with phenotypic expression of a disease. Taken together, RFLPs are very useful as genetic markers for linkage analysis; however, they do quite often suffer from serious drawbacks — one which has already been alluded to is the frequency of nonpolymorphic markers. In addition, the time it takes to complete such an analysis restricts the number of assays that can be achieved in any one week.

2. CA-REPEAT ANALYSIS

More recently, a class of DNA has been identified which relies on a completely different type of polymorphism. There exist, again throughout the genome, repetitive sequences of DNA which can be categorized into the

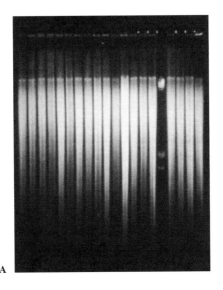

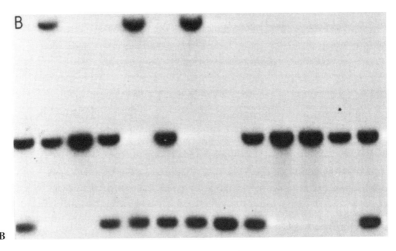

FIGURE 3. A) Fully digested DNA size-fractionated on an agarose gel. B) Representative Southern blot showing the various alleles that are present in the family members who are at risk of having inherited a predisposition to a familial cancer.

following groups: variable number of tandem repeats (VNTRs), which are relatively short nucleotide sequences that are arranged in tandem arrays,[11] and di- and tri-nucleotide repeat sequences which are either doublets or triplets of bases (often referred to as "CA-repeats") dispersed throughout the genome.[12] Most commonly used of these repetitive sequences of DNA are the di- and tri-nucleotide repeats.

Repetitive sequences of DNA are often much more polymorphic than RFLPs and are therefore more useful for linkage analysis. The advantage of CA-repeats is that they can be generated from small amounts of genomic DNA by polymerase chain reaction (PCR). Thereafter, analysis is rapid using acrylamide gel electrophoresis. Depending on the type of CA-repeat, analysis can be performed with or without radioactive tagging of the PCR product (see Figure 4 for examples of both).

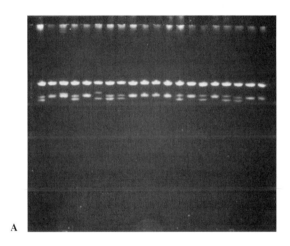

A

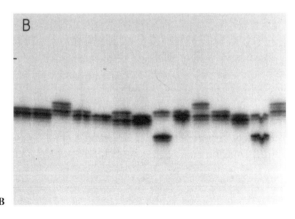

B

FIGURE 4. CA-repeat analysis performed using: A) nonradioactive methods, or B) radioactive methods.

More recently, di- and tri-nucleotide repeat sequences have found another role with respect to familial cancer diagnosis. Thibodeau et al. in 1993 reported that, in certain colorectal carcinomas, expansion and contraction of di- and tri-nucleotide sequences occurred, implying that the underlying genetic defect was associated with a DNA repair deficiency.[13] Examination of di- or tri-nucleotide repeats is identical to that of CA-repeat analysis. For this analysis it is essential to have tumor material from which tumor DNA can be extracted. As it is based on a PCR approach, the amount of material required is minimal. To prove beyond doubt that expansion or contraction of di- or tri-nucleotide repeats is not an artifact of PCR, several different loci throughout the genome should be investigated to ensure that it is a real phenomenon.

Interpretation of either RFLPs or CA-repeats requires the use of a computer to calculate the likelihood of linkage to a particular disease. From such computations, risk assessment can be performed based on the haplotype pattern of the affected individuals within the family. To effectively analyze a family, the phenomenon of crossing-over must be taken into account as this is a relatively frequent event, especially if the markers that are under investigation happen to lie some distance away from the putative gene. Briefly, crossing-over occurs at random, however, there may be sites on a chromosome where the frequency of crossing-over is higher than expected.[14] The result of a cross-over is termed a recombination. Recombinations are extremely useful in positioning a marker with respect to a given gene as they can help to orientate the direction in which a gene lies in relation to the markers used for its identification.

3. Chromosome Analysis

Chromosome analysis has over recent years become more popular for the investigation of genetic differences as it has become possible to combine traditional chromosome analysis with the modern techniques of molecular biology. By far the most important advance that has occurred is the introduction of the fluorescent in situ hybridization technique (FISH) which is based on the following: DNA of interest must be fluorescently tagged such that it can be visualized under UV-light. As this method is specific, it can be used for a number of purposes, such as the detection of an increased copy number of a particular gene or the loss of a piece of DNA from a specific chromosome.[15] The advantage of this technique compared to older methods is that chromosomes can be investigated one at a time; specific chromosome markers are available such that nowadays there is no confusion when determining which chromosome carries the disease allele. Currently this method does not play a major role in direct familial cancer diagnosis but may be used to gain some insight into the prognosis of a person who comes from a family predisposed to disease.

B. DIRECT GENETIC TESTING

Direct genetic testing is only possible when a susceptibility gene has been identified and sequenced. A recent example is that of the adenomatous polyposis coli gene associated with the development of colorectal cancer in persons coming from FAP families. Once a gene has been isolated and sequenced there exists an array of methods which could be used to determine if a mutation lies within it. These shall be dealt with one by one. All the methods described below concerning mutation detection rely on the use of the polymerase chain reaction, which can specifically amplify sequences of interest to amounts that are readily available for analysis.

1. Single Strand Conformation Polymorphism (SSCP) Analysis

This method relies on the conformation of single stranded DNA being a function of the base pair composition of the particular piece of DNA under investigation. In 1989, Orita et al. first described the method whereby DNA is firstly amplified by PCR and then resolved on a nondenaturing acrylamide gel.[16,17] Under these conditions single stranded DNA will form a particular quaternary structure based on its sequence. There are two points that are critical for this method to work effectively. The first is that the DNA should not be more than 400 base pairs in length, any longer and the structure tends to lose its specificity; secondly, only very small amounts of DNA should be applied to the gel as too much causes interaction between the different single stranded DNA species, again leading to a loss of resolution. This method will only be

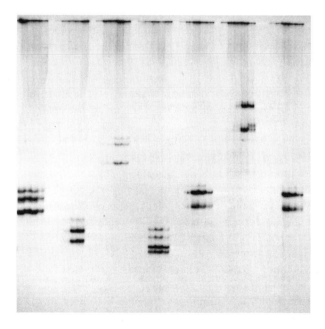

FIGURE 5. An example of a SSCP gel showing various different stretches of DNA that were analyzed by this method. The conformational shifts are indicated by the arrows.

able to distinguish if there is a difference between one single strand and another and it can not be used to definitely determine if a mutation exists in a particular strand of DNA (see Figure 5). Mutation identification can only reliably be performed by sequence analysis, which will be dealt with later. Once a polymorphism is found in an affected person, other members of his or her family should be studied to determine if this polymorphism segregates with the disease. Should it do so, some evidence is provided to support the notion that this polymorphism does indeed represent the site where a mutation in the DNA sequence occurs.

The advantage of this method is that the oligonucleotides can be used both for SSCP and PCR sequencing. The disadvantage is that it requires rather high levels of radioactivity and this can be a problem to some laboratories who do not have adequate disposal facilities. This method can be used to detect approximately 90% of conformational polymorphisms, making it probably the most cost-effective method of mutation detection.[18]

2. Denaturing Gradient Gel Electrophoresis (DGGE)

This is probably the second most common method used for polymorphism detection. It is based on the principle that the annealing temperature of DNA is a function of the base pair composition such that any given double stranded DNA sequence will only under certain specific conditions become single stranded, and that they vary from sequence to sequence.[19] There are two principal methods that can be applied to melt double stranded DNA, the first being temperature, which will be dealt with later, and the second is by increasing the concentration of denaturant (such as urea or formamide). A schematic representation is shown in Figure 6 indicating that sequence A melts at a slightly different concentration of denaturant compared to sequence B.

As the differences between double stranded DNA sequences may not be too obvious using the PCR reaction, a GC tail (of approximately 40 base pairs) can be added to the molecule of interest. This has the advantage of acting as a clamp at one end of the molecule and prevents it from falling apart completely. Under extremely stringent conditions, however, the GC clamp will also come apart and result in a single stranded sequence. This phenomenon of different "melting temperatures" can be utilized during polyacrylamide gel electrophoresis. As the molecule begins to "melt" its migration is retarded, whereas another similar but different sequence will migrate at a faster rate until it too "melts", as shown in Figure 6. In addition, the DNA stain ethidium bromide is more effective when used on double stranded DNA, than single stranded DNA making the addition of the GC clamp more sensitive and thus the procedure more precise. In addition to the homoduplexes observed, there are heteroduplexes present which are formed as a result of heating the DNA prior to application on the gel, which leads to the formation of single stranded DNA that upon reannealing forms double stranded DNA with complementary and noncomplementary sequences, producing homoduplexes and heteroduplexes.

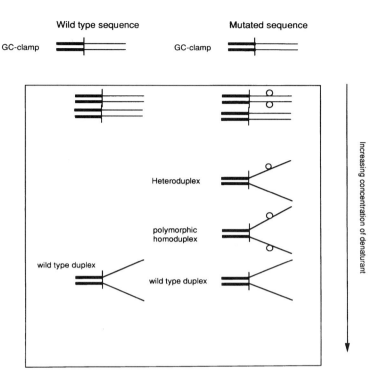

FIGURE 6. Schematic representation of DGGE analysis showing differences in the melting temperature of DNA in a denaturing gradient acrylamide gel. Due to the sequence differences the DNA fragments are retarded in their migration at different denaturant concentrations.

Heteroduplexes often are a source of confusion as they appear to complicate the analysis of polymorphisms. In practice they do not represent much of a problem and in fact help by identifying true polymorphisms when they are difficult to resolve. An example of a DGGE gel is shown in Figure 7; in this example all but one of the samples are identical.

An additional method that is often used for diagnosis is constant gradient gel electrophoresis (CGGE). This method is similar to DGGE, but differs only in the fact that an optimal gradient is chosen for the resolution of the two different DNA sequences.[20] Otherwise the method and its limitations are identical.

The limitation with respect to the size of DNA sequence that can be analyzed is similar to that described for SSCP. The advantage of this method compared to SSCP is that it requires no radioactive marker and is much faster to perform in that no exposure time for autoradiography is required. A difficulty that can be encountered with this method is the development of oligonucleotides used for the PCR reaction. This is due to the fact that the addition of a GC clamp alters the affinity of annealing of the DNA sequence of interest

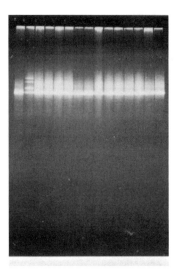

FIGURE 7. A DGGE gel showing the separation of homoduplex DNA from heteroduplex DNA. In this example fifteen different DNA samples were analyzed but only one of them contained a sequence polymorphism.

such that unexpected results may occur. Most of the problems associated with the development of such oligonucleotides can be foreseen using the computer program Melt 87 and SQHTX.[21] Finally, to ensure that the chosen oligonucleotide pair denatures within a certain range of denaturant a two-dimensional gel should be run which will allow the localization of the optimal denaturing concentration. The last and perhaps more important factor for a number of laboratories is the cost, as the GC clamped oligonucleotides not only cost more to produce but also cannot be used in sequence analysis.

3. Temperature Gradient Gel Electrophoresis

Temperature gradient electrophoresis relies essentially on the same principles as DGGE, differing in the one important point that temperature is used instead of a chemical denaturant. The main advantage of this method is that it requires no radioactive tag, therefore eliminating the problems of radioactive waste. The major disadvantage of this technique is that it is extremely difficult to establish the best conditions for each oligonucleotide pair. Due to this reason alone, it is the least favored of the three techniques. In addition, special equipment needs to be obtained for running the resolving gels, as the temperature at which the DNA sequences melt is critical and therefore must be kept absolutely constant throughout the electrophoresis.

4. Mismatch Cleavage Analysis (RNase Protection Assay)

This technique relies on chemical or enzymatic cleavage of mismatches in heteroduplex RNA, causing a break at the site of such differences. Essentially, synthetic complementary RNA must be synthesized that is radioactively labeled which is then hybridized to the RNA sequence under investigation. After hybridization, the heteroduplex is incubated with either RNase A or is chemically cleaved, cutting the resulting hybrid molecule where there is a mismatch in the sequence. Thereafter, the products are applied to a denaturing polyacrylamide gel and resolved by electrophoresis. It appears that RNA mismatch cleavage analysis based on enzymatic analysis is not as sensitive as chemical cleavage such that most workers prefer the chemical cleavage approach even though it requires more effort.[22] RNase protection analysis is currently recognized as being less sensitive than chemical cleavage, which has found more favor recently.[23,24] Both procedures, however, require more steps to complete and do not appear to be as efficient as SSCP or DGGE analysis.

5. Protein/RNA Analysis

Analysis of proteins that have been artificially translated has become useful in the identification of persons at risk suffering from some inherited disorders. Principally, one condition must be fulfilled prior to establishing this technique. The majority of mutations should result in a stop codon such that differences between the mutated and wild type gene product can be clearly seen, as is the case for familial adenomatous polyposis.[25]

Broadly, the aim of the method is to isolate high grade mRNA, translate it in a reticulocyte lysate system, and analyze the protein by sodium dodecyl sulfate-polyacrylamide gel electrophoresis (SDS-PAGE).

The method essentially involves isolation of RNA, which can be achieved by a number of methods such as the guanidinium isothiocyanate method,[26] the lithium chloride method,[27] or the proteinase K digestion method.[28] The major difficulty in working with RNA is in the handling of naked RNA as it is very susceptible to the action of RNases which can rapidly degrade RNA. Therefore, methods need to be employed that contain RNase-inhibiting substances. Thereafter, extreme care must be taken to ensure that the samples do not become contaminated with RNase.

6. Sequencing Analysis

Sequencing analysis is required to establish if different DNA sequences detected with any of the aforementioned methods are in fact mutated sequences that give rise to aberrant gene products or are merely sequence polymorphisms that do not result in any change.

There are essentially two methods by which genes can be sequenced, both of which were developed at approximately the same time. The dideoxy chain termination method developed by Sanger et al.[29] is favored against the chemical sequencing method developed by Maxam and Gilbert.[30] Both methods, however, are based on high resolution denaturing polyacrylamide gel electrophoresis procedures which are capable of resolving single stranded oligodeoxynucleotide sequences of up to 500 base pairs in length that differ in length by a single nucleotide. For a given region of DNA that needs to be sequenced, four different reactions must be performed such that a set of labeled (either radioactive or fluorescent) single stranded oligodeoxynucleotides are generated that are fixed at one end and differ in length at the other end by each successive deoxynucleotide in the sequence. The oligodeoxynucleotides are fixed using a small sequence of DNA that attaches to a known sequence of DNA upstream of the sequence under investigation. Until recently, DNA sequences of interest had to be cloned into suitable plasmid vectors that could then be sequenced using a small compatible plasmid sequence as the anchor site, known as the primer sequence. The key to determining the sequence product is to generate, in four separate chemical or enzymatic reactions, all of the oligodeoxynucleotides that terminate at the variable end in A, T, G, or C, respectively. The products of the four reactions are then resolved electrophoretically under denaturing conditions on a sequencing gel. As all possible oligodeoxynucleotides are represented, a ladder will be generated consisting of all the different sized products.

More recently, direct sequencing reactions can be performed by PCR, where several advantages can be realized.[31] In this instance, the primer sequence which anchors the template DNA is known to be complementary to the sequence of interest. As the PCR reaction is employed, a linear amplification of the DNA sequence under investigation can be performed such that a reduced level of DNA sample is required for sequencing. As the annealing temperature of the template (DNA to be sequenced) is higher using the PCR method, there is an increase in the stringency of primer hybridization which implies greater specificity.

If there are large amounts of sequencing to perform, an alternative automated approach is now possible, which is based on the same principles as those already described. The most prohibitive aspect of automated sequencing is the cost of the apparatus; however, once in use, an automated approach is not only faster but also cheaper than manual methods as it relies on fluorescently labeled bases. This eliminates the need for radioactive nucleotides and with it the problem of radioactive waste disposal.

In summary, sequencing strategies are becoming easier to perform such that familial cancer diagnosis can be performed relatively quickly. Currently, radioactive assays are most often used for analyses that are time-consuming and labor intensive. In the future, more and more groups will start using automated sequencers, which will make this aspect of familial diagnosis more accessible for routine analysis.

IV. CONCLUSION

The methods described here are all associated with the identification of persons at risk of having inherited a genetic predisposition to develop cancer. As an increasing number of genes associated with given diseases are discovered, more emphasis will be placed on the early detection of predisposing genetic factors. With it, new and more rapid methods will be developed for screening purposes such that the identification of persons at risk will become much easier. Unfortunately, associated with increased use of presymptomatic diagnosis is the increase in the likelihood that the results become available to third parties.

REFERENCES

1. **Bishop, D. T. and Thomas, H. J. W.** The genetics of colorectal cancer. *Cancer Surv.* 9, 585, 1990.
2. **Lynch, H. T., Lanspa, S., Smyrk, T., Boman, B., Watson, P., and Lynch, J.** Hereditary nonpolyposis colorectal cancer (Lynch syndromes I & II) *Cancer Genet. Cytogenet.* 53, 143, 1991.
3. **Bülow, S.** Familial polyposis coli. *Dan. Med. Bull.* 34, 1, 1987.
4. **Iselius, L., Slack, J., Littler, M., and Morton, N. E.** Genetic epidemiology of breast cancer in Britain. *Ann. Hum. Genet.* 55, 151, 1991.
5. **Ballabio, A.** The rise and fall of positional cloning, *Nat. Genet.* 3, 277, 1993.
6. **Herrera, L., Kakati, S., Gibas, L., Pietrzak, E., and Sandberg, A. A.** Gardner syndrome in a man with an interstitial deletion of 5q. *Am. J. Med. Genet.* 25, 473, 1986.
7. **Fischel, R., Lescoe, M. K., Rao, M. R. S., Copeland, N. G., Jenkins, N. A., Garber, J., Kane, M., and Kolodner, R.** The human mutator gene homolog MSH2 and its association with hereditary nonpolyposis colon cancer. *Cell* 75, 1027, 1993.
8. **Easton, D. F., Bishop, D. T., Ford, D., Crockford, G. P., and the Breast Cancer Linkage Consortium.** Genetic linkage analysis in familial breast and ovarian cancer. Results from 214 families. *Am. J. Hum. Genet.* 52, 678, 1993.
9. **Lathrop, G. M., Lalouel, J. M., Julier, C., and Ott, J.** Strategies for multilocus linkage analysis in humans. *Proc. Natl. Acad. Sci. U.S.A.* 81, 3443, 1984.
10. **Southern, E. M.** Detection of specific sequences among DNA fragments separated by gel electrophoresis. *J. Mol. Biol.* 98, 503, 1975.
11. **Nakamura, Y., Leppert, M., O'Connell, P., Wolff, R., Holm, T., Culver, M., Martin, C., Fujimoto, E., Hoff, M., Kumlin, E., and White, R.** Variable number of tandem repeat (VNTR) markers for human gene mapping. *Science* 235, 1616, 1987.
12. **Weber, J. L. and May, P. E.** Abundant class of human DNA polymorphisms which can be typed using the polymerase chain reaction. *Am. J. Hum. Genet.* 44, 388, 1989.
13. **Thibodeau, S. N., Bren, G., and Schaid, D.** Microsatellite instability in cancer of the proximal colon. *Science* 269, 816, 1993.
14. **Ott, J.** *Analysis of Human Genetic Linkage*, 2nd ed. Johns Hopkins University Press, Baltimore, 1991.
15. **Cremer, A. J., Lichter, P., Borden, J., Ward, W. C., and Manuelidis, L.** Detection of chromosome aberrations in metaphase and interphase tumor cells by in situ hybridization using chromosome specific library probes. *Hum. Genet.* 85, 235, 1988.
16. **Orita, M., Iwahana, H., Kanazawa, H., Hayashi, K., and Sekiya, T.** Detection of polymorphisms of human DNA by gel electrophoresis as single-strand conformation polymorphisms. *Proc. Natl. Acad. Sci. U.S.A.* 86, 2766, 1989.
17. **Orita, M., Suzuki, Y., Sekiya, T., and Hayashi, K.** Rapid and sensitive detection of point mutations and DNA polymorphisms using the polymerase chain reaction. *Genomics*

5, 874, 1989.

18. **Hayashi, K. and Yandell, D. W.** How sensitive is PCR-SSCP. *Hum. Mutat.* 2, 338, 1993.

19. **Myers, R. M., Maniatis, T., and Lerman, L. S.** Detection and localization of single base changes by denaturing gradient gel electrophoresis. *Methods Enzymol.* 155, 501, 1987.

20. **Borrensen, A.-L., Hovig, E., Smith-Sorensen, B., Malkin, D., Lystad, S., Andersen, T. I., Nesland, J. M., Isselbacher, K. J., and Friend, S. H.** Constant denaturant gel electrophoresis as a rapid screening technique for p53 mutations. *Proc. Natl. Acad. Sci. U.S.A.* 88, 8405, 1991.

21. **Lerman, L. S. and Silverstein, K.** Computational simulation of DNA melting and its application to denaturing gradient gel electrophoresis. *Methods Enzymol.* 155, 482, 1987.

22. **Cotton, R. G. H., Rodrigues, N. R., and Campbell, R. D.** Reactivity of cytosine and thymine in single-base-pair mismatches with hydroxylamine and osmium tetroxide and its application to the study of mutations. *Proc. Natl. Acad. Sci. U.S.A.* 85, 4397, 1988.

23. **Winter, E., Yamamoto, F., Almoguera, C., and Perucho, M.** A method to detect and characterize point mutations in transcribed genes: amplification and overexpression and of the mutant c-K-ras allele in human tumor cells. *Proc. Natl. Acad. Sci. U.S.A.* 82, 7575, 1985.

24. **Myers, R. M., Larin, Z., and Maniatis, T.** Detection of single base substitutions by ribonuclease cleavage at mismatches in RNA:DNA duplex. *Science* 230, 1242, 1985.

25. **Powell, S. W., Petersen, G. M., Krush, A. J., Booker, S., Jen, J., Giardello, F. M., Hamilton, S. R., Vogelstein, B., and Kinzler, K.** Molecular diagnosis of familial adenomatous polyposis. *N. Engl. J. Med.* 329, 1982, 1993.

26. **Chirgwin, J. J., Przbyla, A. E., Macdonald, R. J., and Rutter, W. J.** Isolation of biologically active ribonucleic acid from sources enriched in ribonuclease. *Biochemistry* 18, 5294, 1979.

27. **Berk, A. J. and Sharp, P. A.** Sizing and mapping of early adenovirus mRNAs by gel electrophoresis of S1 endonuclease-digested hybrids. *Cell* 12, 721, 1977.

28. **Palmiter, R. D.** Magnesium precipitation of ribonucleoprotein complexes. Expedient techniques for the isolation of undegraded polysomes and messenger ribonucleic acid. *Biochemistry* 13, 3606, 1974.

29. **Sanger, F., Nicklen, S., and Coulson, A. R.** DNA sequencing with chain terminating inhibitors. *Proc. Natl. Acad. Sci. U.S.A.* 74, 5463, 1977.

30. **Maxam, A. M. and Gilbert, W.** A new method for sequencing DNA. *Proc. Natl. Acad. Sci. U.S.A.* 74, 560, 1977.

31. **Ansorge, W., Sproat, B. S., Stegemann, J., and Schwager, C.** A non-radioactive automated method for DNA sequence determination. *J. Biochem. Biophys. Methods* 13, 315, 1986.

Chapter 8

SURGICAL MANAGEMENT OF FAMILIAL CANCER SYNDROMES

Solange D. MacArthur, Jukka-Pekka Mecklin, and Lemuel Herrera

CONTENTS

I. INTRODUCTION

The following chapter emphasizes the surgical aspects relevant to screening, early detection, and prophylactic and therapeutic interventions in the following clinical syndromes: familial dysplastic nevus syndrome (DNS); multiple endocrine neoplasia type 2 (MEN 2); breast-ovary cancer syndrome (BOCS); hereditary nonpolyposis colon cancer (HNPCC); and familial adenomatous polyposis (FAP).

0-8493-4782-3/96/$0.00+$.50
© 1996 by CRC Press Inc.

II. FAMILIAL DYSPLASTIC NEVUS SYNDROME

Classic familial dysplastic nevus syndrome (DNS), as defined by the Amsterdam group, is characterized by the presence of numerous (often greater than 100) nevi of atypical histology and early onset melanoma.[1] Multiple normal appearing nevi tend to appear in affected patients in childhood, mostly on the trunk and extremities. These nevi increase in number and size throughout puberty, generally developing dysplastic features by early adulthood.[2,3] The term "dysplastic" when applied to these lesions may be used to describe more than one histological pattern: melanocytic hypertrophy, lateral junctional melanocytic proliferation with cellular atypia, junctional or compound melanocytic nevi with architectural atypia, and/or cytological atypia are just a few of the descriptive morphological terms used.[3,4] Grossly, the dysplastic nevus is larger than ordinary nevi, has an ill-defined border which tends to merge subtly into normal skin, and appears macular with pinkish, irregular coloration.[3,5] Although progression of dysplasia to malignancy is not obligatory, it has been well documented in the familial syndrome.[6-9] Classic familial dysplastic nevus syndrome confers to individuals at risk a lifetime chance of developing cutaneous melanoma several hundred times greater than individuals from the general population.[5]

Surgical management of patients identified with, or suspected of DNS focuses on prevention of melanoma by identification and removal of the dysplastic nevi. Programs for screening and early detection should include photographic or video documentation of all body surfaces and examinations with detailed measurements of the lesions every 3 to 6 months.[3,10,11] Patient and family education should be comprehensive: self-examination teaching, risk assessment for patients and their families, genetic counseling, and enrollment into follow-up registries are of paramount importance in the multidisciplinary management of DNS, especially now that there is the possibility of having the melanoma-associated gene mutations localized to chromosome 9p13-22.

Clinically dysplastic, new, or changing nevi should be excised with a narrow margin (1–3 mm) to exclude malignant transformation.[2,5] This approach has minimized diagnostic problems and the lesion's evolution into melanoma.[3,12-14] "Shave" biopsies are to be discouraged as this procedure distorts measurement of linear depth should the lesion turn out to be a melanoma.[3] Nevi in areas of the body difficult to observe, e.g., scalp and other hairy areas, anus, and umbilicus, should be excised prophylactically.[2]

Once melanoma is diagnosed in the context of DNS, it is managed in the same way as sporadic cases, as the prognostic factors and course of disease do not differ.[6,7] Patients with DNS may have melanoma diagnosed at an earlier stage due to intensive surveillance.

III. MULTIPLE ENDOCRINE NEOPLASIA TYPE 2

MEN 2a and 2b are autosomal dominantly inherited cancer syndromes with a high degree of penetrance characterized by medullary thyroid cancer (MTC) and pheochromocytoma. MEN 2a is associated with hyperparathyroidism in 20 to 30% of patients while MEN 2b is distinguished by the presence of submucosal ganglioneuromas and a marfanoid habitus. Although pheochromocytomas are life-threatening tumors in the acute setting, MTC remains the major cause of death in affected individuals.

Medullary thyroid cancer or its precursor lesion, C-cell hyperplasia, has been found in nearly 100% of studied individuals with MEN 2.[17-18] Screening by family history and DNA linkage analysis, combined with repetitive provocative testing for abnormal calcitonin response, has been used to select patients with MEN 2a for prophylactic thyroidectomy.[19,20] MEN 2b patients identified by their distinctive phenotype have been candidates for early prophylactic total thyroidectomy without the usual provocative calcitonin testing practiced for MEN 2a.[21] MTC is an aggressive cancer and has been found in affected patients in early childhood, even in the absence of abnormal calcitonin stimulation.[22] Early total thyroidectomy, possibly in infancy, is recommended by some authors.[23,24] Wells et al.[29] reported no evidence of metastatic spread in 10 MEN 2a patients aged 6 to 20 years who were identified by molecular biology and underwent total thyroidectomy for clinically occult MTC (T0 N0 M0). They feel that thyroidectomy should be performed on MEN 2a patients from the age of 5 years, with a curative or preventive intent.[29]

A number of germline missense mutations in the RET protooncogene have been found in individuals with MEN 2a and 2b.[25-28] Recent reports on the effectiveness of DNA testing to detect RET mutations in MEN 2a may have all but eliminated the need for provocative testing for early detection of MTC. Just as importantly, DNA testing in MEN 2 kindreds should eliminate the need for lifelong biochemical screening in noncarriers of the MEN 2 gene.[29,30]

Total thyroidectomy in MEN 2a or b should include central lymph node dissection. Modified radical neck dissection is added in the presence of known carcinoma or a palpable neck mass.[31] Larimore and Wells, at Washington University, reported a 13% MTC recurrence rate for asymptomatic, biochemically detected disease, as opposed to 58% recurrence for tumors detected by physical exam.[19] More recently, Wells' group described the surgical strategy of total thyroidectomy, total parathyroidectomy, and central lymph node dissection with autotransplantation of parathyroid tissue to the nondominant forearm for all asymptomatic MEN 2a gene carriers.[29] Serum calcium was normal without supplementation 10 weeks after surgery for all 13 patients in this series.

There is a subset of MEN 2 patients diagnosed with concurrent pheochromocytoma and medullary thyroid cancer or C-cell hyperplasia. These patients may undergo either a one-stage procedure or surgery in two stages. Pheochromocytomas are always resected first, after appropriate preoperative blood pressure control. Young, healthy patients may be better served by resection of pheochromocytoma, followed by total thyroidectomy under the same anesthesia. Hospital stay may be significantly decreased with this approach, with no increased morbidity or mortality.[32] However, most patients have first undergone separate resection of the pheochromocytoma, with thyroidectomy later in the same hospitalization.

A. PHEOCHROMOCYTOMA

The presence of pheochromocytoma is an indication for a surgical resection. These patients are at significant risk for sudden death. Pheochromocytomas behave similarly in MEN 2a and 2b and are managed in the same way.

In general, while most patients with sporadic pheochromocytoma present with a history and symptoms consistent with the diagnosis, MEN 2 patients in screening programs may be diagnosed before the onset of symptomatic disease by determination of urine catecholamines and their metabolites. Approximately 50% of MEN 2 patients develop pheochromocytoma,[20] of whom 50 to 90% will have bilateral tumors diagnosed, synchronously or metachronously.[33-35] Bilateral pheochromocytomas are resected at the same operation via an anterior approach and a careful examination of the aortic paraganglia performed. There is sharp division between authors in the field over whether bilateral adrenalectomy should be performed in MEN 2 patients in whom one adrenal gland appears grossly normal at surgery for unilateral pheochromocytoma. Advocates of unilateral adrenalectomy in such cases cite a low incidence of malignancy and high incidence of complications associated with the hypoadrenal state. A significant number of MEN 2 patients presenting with unilateral pheochromocytoma will take years to develop a second tumor, allowing them a longer period of life uncomplicated by the risks of long-standing steroid maintenance therapy or Addisonian crisis.[20,34,35] Second surgery via a posterior (retroperitoneal) approach is well tolerated for a documented tumor in the remaining gland. Proponents of preemptive bilateral adrenalectomy in all MEN 2 patients with pheochromocytoma dispute the existence of significant problems with long-term steroid replacement therapy, emphasize the almost universal microscopic finding of abnormal medullary cells in the contralateral adrenal gland, and the high likelihood of second surgery required in the future.[36-38] The incidence of malignant pheochromocytoma in MEN 2 patients is low,[33,39,40] however, patients with a family history of malignant pheochromocytoma should be considered for bilateral adrenalectomy, even when only unilateral disease is apparent.[35,37,39] Thus, knowledge of the phenotypic neoplastic expression of the kindred, age at diagnosis, patient commitment to compliance, and patient education are important factors influencing a clinical decision.

B. HYPERPARATHYROIDISM

Primary hyperparathyroidism in MEN 2a is less prevalent and tends to be milder than in MEN 1.[41] Hyperparathyroidism is not part of the MEN 2b syndrome.[21] Nevertheless, symptomatic disease in MEN 2a patients is not unknown and parathyroidectomy is carried out for all patients meeting criteria for hyperparathyroidism.[42]

Two studies have shown that a conservative surgical approach is warranted in MEN 2a-associated hyperparathyroidism.[41,43] Recurrence was found to be extremely low regardless of the operation performed — subtotal parathyroidectomy, total parathyroidectomy with autotransplantation, or resection of clinically enlarged glands only. In light of the breakthroughs in identifying MEN 2 gene carriers, leading to a surgical strategy of early preemptive total thyroidectomy with autotransplantation of parathyroid tissue, the issue of conservative management of hyperparathyroidism has become less relevant. All four parathyroids should be identified during thyroidectomy with autografting of parathyroid tissue into the muscle of the nondominant forearm. Cryopreservation of extra parathyroid tissue should be done to provide an option if the first graft fails.[44]

IV. SURGICAL MANAGEMENT OF BREAST AND OVARIAN CANCER SYNDROME

With the recent publication of data out of the University of Utah, genetic researchers appear to have identified the gene *BRCA1*, mapped to the chromosome region 17q12-21 and thought responsible for early onset breast-ovarian cancer syndrome.[45] *BRCA1* is believed to be a tumor suppressor gene, thus most women are born with two healthy copies of the gene and have a 12% lifetime risk of developing breast cancer. However, women born with a defective copy of the gene appear to have an 85% risk of developing breast cancer during their lives.[51] Patients identified as carriers of defective *hMSH2* and *hMLH1* are at significant risk for the development of ovarian cancer as well. Another breast cancer susceptibility gene, *BRCA2*, has recently been localized to chromosome 13q.[46] Counseling based on genetic linkage analysis is already available from some groups involved in cancer family research,[47] and, presumably, genetic testing for individuals at risk will become available within the next few years.

There are differences in approach, as well as overlap in opinion, regarding the role of prophylactic surgery in this syndrome.[48,49] Identification of tissues at risk depends on meticulous ascertainment of disease genealogy including age-onset of the disease. Only documented invasive tumors must be included in the family history for analysis. There is overlap between several separate cancer family syndromes as identified by clustering of the disease (e.g., hereditary breast cancer — HBC, hereditary breast-ovarian cancer syndrome — HBOC, Lynch II syndrome).[50,51] As genetic testing for specific *BRCA1* mutations and other cancer protooncogenes becomes widely available, screening of HBOC family members will be carried out quickly and reliably.

Breast carcinoma appears more frequently and generally at a younger decade than ovarian cancer in breast-ovary cancer families; the average age for breast cancer is 45–47, and the mean age for ovarian cancer is 50.[52-55] While screening for breast cancer in the general population is well established and has been shown to be of benefit for women over the age of 40,[56] in women from breast-ovarian cancer syndrome families, intensive screening is recommended as early as age 20 and should include a monthly breast self exam, a physical exam by a physician every 6 months, periodic mammography and/or breast ultrasound (every 1–2 years) from age 25, and yearly mammography from age 35.[48,57] While the value of such screening is still not established, it is clear that patient education is paramount for the success of this approach. Breast ultrasonography is a useful adjunct to a physical exam in young women with dense breast tissue and equivocal findings, for whom mammography is of limited value.[57,58] We have used this diagnostic modality, often in conjunction with fine needle aspirate (FNA) or core biopsy, increasingly over the past several years.

In the general population, breast-conserving surgery with radiation therapy has proven effective, with local control and overall survival results comparable to modified radical mastectomy for early invasive cancer.[59,60] These data, however, have yet to be applied to the subset of patients with inherited breast cancer syndromes.[48] These patients often have bilateral, multicentric tumors; they are emotionally wrought, and cancer phobia may be significant. Although, in theory one could agree with modified radical mastectomy (MRM) for small invasive cancers and total mastectomy for ductal carcinoma *in situ* (DCIS) for most female obligate carriers of *BRCA1* or *BRCA2* mutations, we would recommend an ipsilateral mastectomy, and discuss possible contralateral pro-phylactic mastectomy. Some limited experiences are already available on prophylactic surgery.[61,62] Such a surgical approach is best carried out in close coordination with a team that includes plastic surgery, rehabilitation, and medical oncology and peer support groups, but must be preceded by thorough patient and family preparation in terms of expectations by a clinical oncology geneticist. Chemoprophylaxis with tamoxifen in this clinical setting is of yet unknown benefit.[49,63]

Screening for ovarian cancer has a lower yield for early detection than for breast cancer. Current screening protocols include a 6- to 12-month periodic pelvic physical exam, transvaginal sonography, a Doppler color flow study, and serial CA 125 assays.[48] Each one of these examinations has its strong and weak points, and trials using various combinations are underway.[64-66] Most authors in the field agree that a preemptive bilateral oophorectomy with or without hysterectomy should be performed in HBOC relatives at risk after childbearing is complete, or at least by age 40.[48,57,64] This is especially true for gene carriers of *BRCA1*, *hMSH2*, or *hMLH1* mutations. One must remember that despite preemptive oophorectomy, 5 to 10% of women in this group may still develop a papillary carcinoma arising from peritoneal surfaces and embryonic Muellerian rests, limiting (at least in this group) the value of preemptive therapeutic intervention.[67,68] Low-dose estrogen replacement for these patients, with or without cyclical progesterone, is controversial given their risk for breast cancer. Tamoxifen therapy due to its weak estrogen-like effects on bone loss and cardiovascular disease, has theoretical but unproven advantages.[69-71]

Clearly, because of the complexity of treatment options as well as the emotional issues faced by patients with hereditary breast and ovarian cancer syndrome, they will be best served by a multidisciplinary team with an understanding of hereditary neoplastic disease. These families should be seen first by the clinical geneticist, with surgeons playing a technical supportive role in their management.

V. HEREDITARY NONPOLYPOSIS COLORECTAL CANCER

Identification of hereditary nonpolyposis colon cancer (HNPCC) families has relied on detailed disease genealogies of patients presenting with early onset (mean age 45) colon carcinoma as dictated by the Amsterdam criteria.[1,72] Recently, two genes, *hMSH2* (2p) and *hMLH1* (3p) have been implicated in the pathogenesis of HNPCC in some kindreds, allowing for the possibility of detecting gene carriers in individuals at risk.[73-76] These two genes seem to account for a major share of HNPCC,[77] however, two additional gene mutations, *hPMS1* and *hPMS2*, have recently been found in some HNPCC patients.[78]

Current recommendations for screening in HNPCC families consist of colonoscopy, or air-contrast barium enema combined with flexible proctosigmoidoscopy (64 cm). Flat adenomas, the putative premalignant lesion, are best recognized at colonoscopy by an experienced clinician familiar with these lesions. These studies are begun between the ages of 20 and 25 years. Evaluation of the colon is performed yearly: if two consecutive colonoscopies are found to be normal, examination is repeated every 3 years or for evaluation of colonic symptoms.[55]

Patients with hereditary nonpolyposis colorectal cancer require a more extensive surgical procedure than those with sporadic colorectal cancer. As HNPCC can be associated with a number of extracolonic neoplastic manifestations, prophylactic resection of other target organs, e.g., ovaries, may become an issue in kindreds expressing neoplastic phenotypes.

Lynch et al. reported an 18.1% incidence of synchronous colon cancers and 24.2% metachronous colon cancers in HNPCC.[79,80] Mecklin and Jarvinen reported a disturbingly high incidence of second colon cancers within 3 years in HNPCC patients who had undergone segmental resections of their original tumor.[81] They observed a 50% chance for the development of a second colorectal cancer and a 20% chance of a third colorectal cancer within 10 years. Thus, for patients identified with HNPCC we recommend subtotal colectomy with ileorectal anastomosis when a cancer is found, or when multiple diffuse flat adenoma are documented.[82] Although abdominal colectomy with a colonic reservoir has been suggested, long-term follow-up in these patients is not known.[83] Preservation of a colon reservoir would theoretically decrease morbidity related to frequent stools, while maintaining easy access for subsequent surveillance with the 64 cm flexible proctosigmoidoscope. We do not favor a colonic reservoir, as we see little benefit but potentially significant risks.

A number of other malignancies are associated with HNPCC. Lifetime risks have been estimated at 20% for endometrial cancer, 12% for urinary tract and gastric cancers, and 6% for ovarian cancer.[84,85] The risk of biliopancreatic and small bowel adenocarcinoma is also significantly increased in HNPCC.[86-88] Prophylactic total abdominal hysterectomy with bilaterial salphigoophorectomy (TAH-BSO) becomes an important consideration in women undergoing abdominal surgery for colon cancer. In this clinical setting, we would recommend that TAH-BSO is combined with colectomy for women over the age of 40, when childbearing has been completed, or in obligate gene carriers of *hMSH2*, *hMLH1*, or *BRCA1*.

VI. SURGICAL MANAGEMENT OF FAMILIAL ADENOMATOUS POLYPOSIS

Familial adenomatous polyposis (FAP) is characterized by multiple (usually over 100) colonic polyps of mixed histology, but predominantly adenomatous in nature. Polyps are usually diagnosed at a median age of 16 years (range: 5–38). Without intervention, patients with this syndrome have a 100% chance of developing invasive colon adenocarcinoma arising from one of the polyps. Colectomy of varying extent has been the mainstay in the management of FAP. A number of extracolonic neoplasms, benign and malignant, are associated with FAP, some of which are also best managed surgically.

Extensively described and well recognized as a familial cancer syndrome, familial adenomatous polyposis provided a framework for the establishment of a registry. In 1985, the Leeds Castle Polyposis Group was founded as a result of an international meeting of FAP workers held in Leeds Castle, England. This group, comprised of 19 centers worldwide, was formed with the main goals of: documenting worldwide incidence; describing geographical differences in phenotype; creating a clinical clearing house, i.e., patient registries; establishing age-onset of phenotypical manifestations; following trends of treatment; coordinating research protocols; validating the efficacy of predictive testing; and educating patients and relatives at risk.[89,90]

The establishment of patient and family registries has been the cornerstone of advancing knowledge in the field of familial adenomatous polyposis, as well as in other cancer family syndromes.

The value of hereditary cancer registries cannot be overly stressed. Patient and family education combined with the continuity of follow-ups have clearly led to decreased mortality from colorectal cancer due to FAP in enrolled families.[91] With the advent of DNA testing to reliably identify those family members at risk, these registries will become even more effective in the coordination of research, care, and education of family members specifically at risk.

Genetic diagnosis of FAP has recently become a reality with the identification of the adenomatous polyposis coli (*APC*) gene.[92] As with *BRCA1*, this gene is large, with over 300,000 base pairs, and the sequences encoding the APC protein are separated in 15 pieces or exons. The APC protein is comprised of 2,843 amino acids with a mass of 300 kDa. Some of the differences in clinical characteristics may be attributable to the nature of the mutations. Although not perfect, practical methods of genetic screening are now applicable to affected families.[93,94] This has led to more specific guidelines in colonoscopic assessment of family members at risk and reducing the need for intensive screening in those not carrying APC mutations.

Patients with FAP are at high risk for a number of other neoplastic manifestations. A brief discussion of the more common associated disorders follows.

A. UPPER GASTROINTESTINAL DISEASE

Upper gastrointestinal polyps are a common finding in patients with FAP. Gastric, duodenal, ampullary, and small-bowel polyps may be identified in over 40% of patients diagnosed with FAP.[91] The large majority of these tumors are benign; however, close follow-up with biopsy is recommended.

Gastric polyps are usually a result of fundic hyperplasia and follow a benign course. However, adenomatous changes with progression to carcinoma *in situ* have also been documented. These polyps are usually flat, sessile, and not amenable to endoscopic resection. They are followed endoscopically, with biopsy. Surgical removal is indicated for symptomatic disease, or biopsy proven dysplasia, or carcinoma *in situ*.[95]

Duodenal and ampullary polyps are more often adenomatous in nature and carry a higher risk of malignant transformation. These polyps are usually small and amenable to endoscopic resection. Polyps not resectable by endoscopic means should be biopsied periodically. Ampullary carcinoma, although rare, is the most common malignancy of the upper gastrointestinal tract experienced by patients with FAP.[91,96] The standard Whipple procedure has a high curative result in closely followed patients.

B. DESMOID TUMORS

Desmoid tumors feature prominently in some families with FAP. These locally invasive, nonmetastasizing soft tissue tumors can develop anywhere in the body. Death from these tumors eventually results from local invasion of critical organ systems. Most problematical desmoids of the bowel mesentery often render surgical resection of bowel carcinoma difficult. Operation of desmoid tumors is reserved for symptomatic disease, as surgery seems to exacerbate regrowth. A number of chemotherapeutic regimens have shown promise in slowing or arresting desmoid growth. Although studies are small in numbers, drugs reported in the treatment of desmoid tumors include sulindac, tamoxifen, and various combinations of cancer chemo-therapeutic agents.[97-100]

C. THYROID DISEASE

Papillary cancer of the thyroid is a relatively uncommon malignancy associated with FAP, but with increased incidence over the general population.[101] Various forms of benign thyroiditis have also been detected in FAP registry-enrolled patients.[102] We recommend total thyroidectomy when cancer is detected, diminishing possible confusion between benign and malignant states and facilitating follow-up.

D. COLONIC SURGERY OPTIONS

Total abdominal colectomy with ileorectal anastomosis is the most common surgical procedure for treatment of FAP. Objection by some of the American authors to this operation is the risk of carcinoma developing in the rectal remnant if patient compliance with lifelong periodic proctoscopy is less than diligent. Advantages of this procedure include a low incidence of sexual impotence, relatively normal bowel function, normal bladder function, and absence of a stoma. The rectal remnant is easily accessible for surveillance and biopsy or polypectomy when required. Orally administered sulindac and difluoromethylornithine have been associated with regression of rectal polyps, but are at this time still in clinical trials.[103-106] Polypectomy or polyp ablation by electro or laser vaporization has been the standard approach.

Total abdominal colectomy with mucosal proctectomy and ileal pouch-anal anastomosis has become increasingly popular for the treatment of ulcerative colitis. Its use has been successfully applied to FAP when reserved for patients with large numbers of rectal polyps without evidence of invasive carcinoma or mesenteric desmoid tumors.[107,108] In experienced hands, this operation eliminates all colorectal tissue at risk for carcinoma while avoiding a stoma, maintaining sphincter control, and usually sparing sexual function.[109] This surgery is difficult and is associated with a higher complication rate than subtotal colectomy. Complications include anastomotic breakdown, small bowel obstruction, incontinence, sexual dysfunction, anastomotic stricture, and pouchitis.[110]

Total proctocolectomy with ileostomy remains a very reasonable surgical option in selected patients with FAP. This procedure's main disadvantage is a permanent stoma which carries well-recognized social, psychological, and stomal skin complications. Nevertheless, proctocolectomy with ileostomy is the procedure of choice for patients who have not tolerated ileoanal anastomosis, the elderly, or those with poor sphincter tone, and patients for whom reliable follow-up is in question.

Segmental resection is rarely indicated in FAP. Patients with metastatic cancer and local tumor complications such as bleeding or obstruction are candidates for minimal resection. Risks vs. benefits must be weighed in resectable, but very high surgical risk patients.

VII. SUMMARY

As reliable genetic testing becomes more available and applicable to a greater number of hereditary cancer syndromes, genetic-directed screening will become a widespread reality. Already, as in the case of MEN 2, a significant impact on the natural history of the disease can be made. The surgical management in this group of patients is altered by knowledge of the stratification of patients as gene carriers, of specific mutations associated to specific phenotypical manifestations, and of the natural history of disease in affected and nonaffected individuals.

The role of hereditary cancer family registries has become invaluable. Genetic counseling and family education have led to a more proactive involvement by patients in their overall care. Extent of surgery, both prophylactic and with curative intent, has been largely based on registry data. Screening protocols have been established and can be expected to become more focused as genetic diagnosis is refined. Preemptive surgery, lifesaving in many cases, will also continue to become more directed. Difficult issues such as patient privacy, emotional impact of early diagnosis, decisions on timing of surgery, and many others, are best taken on by a multidisciplinary team dedicated to the comprehensive care of this special group of patients.

REFERENCES

1. The Netherlands Foundation on the Detection of Hereditary Tumors. Annual Report, 1993, p18.
2. **Tucker, M. A., Greene, M. H., and Clark, W. H.** Dysplastic nevi on the scalp of prepubertal children from melanoma-prone families. *J. Pediatr.* 103: 65–69, 1983.
3. **Crutcher, W. A.** The dysplastic nevus and its clinical management. *Adv. Dermatol.* 3: 187–204, 1988.
4. **Seywright, M. M., Doherty, V. R., and MacKie, R. M.** Proposed alterative terminology and subclassification of so-called "dysplastic nevi". *J. Clin. Pathol.* 39: 189–194, 1986.
5. **Rhodes, A. R.** Potential precursors of cutaneous melanoma. In *Malignant Melanoma: Medical and Surgical Management.* Lejeune, F. J., Chaudhuri, P. K., and Gupta, T. K., Eds. McGraw-Hill, 1994.
6. **Reimer, R. R., Clark, W. H., Jr., Greene, M. H., et al.** Precursor lesions in familial melanoma: A new genetic preneoplastic syndrome. *JAMA.* 239: 744–746, 1978.
7. **Lynch, H. T., Fusaro, R. M., Danes, B. S., et al.** A review of hereditary malignant melanoma including biomarkers in familial atypical multiple mole-melanoma syndrome. *Cancer Genet. Cytogenet.* 8: 325–358, 1983.

8. **Greene, M. H., Clark, W. H., Tucker, M. A., et al.** High risk of malignant melanoma in melanoma prone families with dysplastic nevi. *Ann. Intern. Med.* 102: 458–465, 1985.

9. **Lober, C. W.** Dysplastic (atypical) nevI: Significance and management. *South. Med. J.* 85: 870–887, 1992.

10. **MacKie, R. M., McHenry, P., and Hole, D.** Accelerated detection with prospective surveillance for cutaneous malignant melanoma in high-risk groups. *Lancet* 341(8861): 1618–20, 1993.

11. **Slue, W. E., Jr.** Total body photography for melanoma surveillance. *N.Y. State J. Med.* 92: 494–495, 1992.

12. **Regel, D. S. and Friedman, R. J.** The management of patients with dysplastic and congenital nevi. *Dermatol. Clin.* 3: 251–255, 1985.

13. **Sagebiel, R. W.** Histopathology of borderline and early malignant melanomas. *Am. J. Surg. Pathol.* 3: 543–552, 1979.

14. **Ackerman, A. B. and Mihara, I.** Dysplasia, dysplastic melanaocytes, dysplastic nevi, the dysplastic nevus syndrome, and the relation between dysplastic nevi and malignant melanomas. *Hum. Pathol.* 16: 87–91, 1985.

15. **Ronan, S. G., Han, M. C., and Das Gupta, T. K.** Histologic prognostic indicators in cutaneous malignant melanoma. *Semin. Oncol.* 15: 558–565, 1988.

16. **Hieken, T. J., Rauth, S., Ronan, S. G., et al.** Hereditary melanoma. *Surg. Oncol. Clin. North Am.* 3: 563–577, 1994.

17. **Easton, D. F., Ponder, M. A., and Cummings, T., et al.** The clinical and screening age-at-onset distribution for the MEN-2 syndrome. *Am. J. Hum. Genet.* 44: 208–215, 1989.

18. **Decker, R. A.** Long-term follow-up of a large North American kindred with multiple endocrine neoplasia type 2a. *Surgery* 112: 1066–1073, 1992.

19. **Lairmore, T. C. and Wells, S. A.** Medullary carcinoma of the thyroid: current diagnosis and management. *Semin. Surg. Oncol.* 7: 92–99, 1991.

20. **Gagel, R. F., Tashjian, A. H., Cummings, T., et al.** The clinical outcome of prospective screening for multiple endocrine neoplasia type 2a. An 18-year experience. *N. Engl. J. Med.* 318: 478–484.

21. **Sizemore, G. W., Carney, J. A., Gharib, H., et al.** Multiple endocrine neoplasia type 2b: eighteen-year follow-up of a four-generation family. *Henry Ford Hosp. Med. J.* 40: 236–244, 1992.

22. **Delius, R. E. and Thompson, N. W.** Early total thyroidectomy in patients with multiple endocrine neoplasia 2B syndrome. *Surg. Gynocol. Obstet.* 169: 442–444, 1989.

23. **Telander, R. L., Zimmerman, D., Sizemore, G. W., et al.** Medullary thyroid carcinoma in children. Results of early detection and surgery. *Arch. Surg.* 124: 841–843, 1989.

24. **Samaan, N. A., Draznin, M. B., Halpin, R. E., et al.** Multiple endocrine syndrome type 2b in early childhood. *Cancer* 68: 1832–4, 1991.

25. **Mulligan, L. M., Kwok, J. B., Healey, C. S., et al.** Germ-line mutations of the RET proto-oncogene in multiple endocrine neoplasia type 2A. *Nature* 363 363: 458–460, 1993.

26. **Donis-Keller, H., Dou, S., Chi, D., et al.** Mutations in the RET proto-oncogene are associated with MEN 2A and FMTC. *Hum. Mol. Genet.* 2: 851–856, 1993.

27. **Hofstra, R. M., Landsvater, R. M., Ceccherini, I., et al.** A mutation in the RET proto-oncogene associated with multiple endocrine neoplasia type 2B and sporadic medullary thyroid carcinoma. *Nature* 367 367: 375–376, 1994.

28. **Eng, C., Smith, D. P., Mulligan, L. M., et al.** Point mutation within the tyrosine kinase domain of the RET proto-oncogene in multiple endocrine neoplasia type 2B and related sporadic tumours. *Hum. Mol. Genet.* 3: 237–241, 1994.

29. **Wells, S. A., Jr., Chi, D. D., Toshima, K., et al.** Predictive DNA testing and prophylactic thyroidectomy in patients at risk for multiple endocrine neoplasia type 2A. *Ann. Surg.* 220: 237–250, 1994.

30. **Lips, C. J. M., Landsvater, R. M., Hoppener, J. W. M., et al.** Clinical screening as

compared with DNA analysis in families with multiple endocrine neoplasia type 2a. *N. Engl. J. Med.* 331: 828–835.

31. **Russell, C. F., Van Heerden, J. A., Sizemore, G. W., et al.** The surgical management of medullary thyroid carcinoma. *Ann. Surg.* 197: 42–8, 1983.

32. **Scheumann, G. F. and Dralle, H.** Surgical approach of synchronous medullary thyroid carcinoma and pheochromocytoma in MEN 2 syndrome. *Henry Ford Hosp. Med. J.* 40: 278–280, 1992.

33. **Casanova, S., Rosenberg-Bourgin, M., Farkas, D., et al.** Phaeochromocytoma in multiple endocrine neoplasia type 2 A: survey of 100 cases. *Clin. Endocrinol.* 38: 531–7, 1993.

34. **Fraker, D. L. and Norton, J. A.** Controversies in surgical therapy for APUDomas. *Semin. Surg. Oncol.* 9: 437–442.

35. **Lairmore, T. C., Ball, D. W., Baylin, S. B., and Wells, S. A.** Management of pheochromocytomas in patients with multiple endocrine neoplasia type 2 syndromes. *Ann. Surg.* 217: 595–603, 1993.

36. **Carney, J. A., Sizemore, G. W., and Tyce, G. M.** Bilateral adrenal medullary hyperplasia in multiple endocrine neoplasia, type 2: the precursor of bilateral pheochromocytoma. *Mayo Clin Proc.* 50: 3–10, 1975.

37. **Van Heerden, J. A., Sizemore, G. W., Carney, J. A., et al.** Surgical management of the adrenal glands in the multiple endocrine neoplasia type II syndrome. *World J. Surg.* 8: 612–621, 1984.

38. **Lips, K. J., Van der Sluys Veer, J., Struybenberg, A., et al.** Bilateral occurrence of pheochromocytoma in patients with the multiple endocrine neoplasia syndrome type 2A (Sipple's syndrome). *Am. J. Med.* 70: 1051–60, 1981.

39. **Sisson, J. C., Shapiro, B., and Beierwaltes, W. H.** Scintigraphy with I-131 MIGB as an aid to the treatment of pheochromocytomas in patients with the multiple endocrine neoplasia type 2 syndromes *Henry Ford Hosp. Med. J.* 32: 254–261, 1984.

40. **Melicow, M. M.** One hundred cases of pheochromocytoma (107 tumors) aT the Columbia-Presbyterian Medical Center, 1926–1976. A clinicopathological analysis. *Cancer* 40: 1987–2004, 1977.

41. **O'Riordain, D. S., O'Brian, T., Grant, C. S., et al.** Surgical management of primary hyperparathyroidism in multiple endocrine neoplasia types 1 and 2. *Surgery* 114: 1031–1039, 1993.

42. **Van Heerden, J. A. and Grant, C. S.** Surgical treatment of hyperparathyroidism: an institutional perspective. *World J. Surg.* 15: 688–92, 1991.

43. **Cance, W. G. and Wells, S. A.** Multiple endocrine neoplasia type 2a. *Curr. Probl. Surg.* 22:1, 1985.

44. **van Heerden, J. A., Kent, R. B., III, Sizemore, G. W., et al.** Primary hyperparathyroidism in patients with multiple endocrine neoplasia syndromes. Surgical experience. *Arch. Surg.* 118: 533–6, 1983.

45. **Miki, Y., Swensen, J., Shattuck-Eidens, D., et al.** A strong candidate for breast and ovarian cancer susceptibility gene BRCA 1. *Science* 266: 66–71, 1994.

46. **Wooster, R., Neuhansen, S. L., Nangion, J., et al.** Localization of a breast cancer susceptibility gene, BRCA2, to chromosome 13q12-13. *Science* 265: 2088–2090, 1994.

47. **Biesecker, B. B., Boehnke, M., Calzone, K., et al.** Genetic counseling for families with inherited susceptibility to breast and ovarian cancer. *JAMA* 269: 1970–1974.

48. **Lynch, H. T., Lynch, J., Conway, T., et al.** Hereditary breast cancer and family cancer syndromes. *World J. Surg.* 18: 21–31, 1994.

49. **King, M. C., Rowel, S., and Love, S. M.** Inherited breast and ovarian cancer. *JAMA* 269(15): 1975–1980, 1993.

50. **Hoskins, I. A. and Hoskins, W. J.** Hereditary ovarian cancer. *Surg. Oncol. Clin. North Am.* 3: 523–543, 1994.

51. **Lynch, H. T., Fitzgibbons, R. J., Jr., and Lynch, J. F.** Heterogeneity and natural history of hereditary breast cancer. *Surg. Clin. North Am.* 70: 753–774, 1990.

52. **Easton, D. F., Bishop, D. T., Ford, D., et al.** Genetic linkage analysis in familial breast and ovarian cancer: reslults from 214 families. *Am. J. Hum. Genet.* 52: 678–701, 1993.

53. **Bewtra, C., Watson, P., Conway, T., et al.** Hereditary ovarian cancer: a clinicopathological study. *Int. J. Gynecol. Pathol.* 11: 180–187, 1992.

54. **Vasen, H. F. A., Beex, L. V. A. M., Cleton, F. J., et al.** Clinical heterogeneity of hereditary breast cancer and its impact on screening protocols, the Dutch experience on 24 families under surveillance. *Eur. J. Cancer* 29: 1111–1114, 1993.

55. **Vasen, H. F. A.** Inherited forms of colorectal, breast, ovarian cancer: guidelines for surveillance. *Surg. Oncol. Clin. North Am.* 3: 501–521, 1994.

56. **NCI.** Breast Screening Consortium; screening mammography: a missed opportunity. *JAMA* 4: 54, 1990.

57. **Cruickshank, D. J., Haites, N., Anderson, S., et al.** The multidisciplinary management of a family with epithelial ovarian cancer. *Br. J. Obstet. Gynaecol.* 99: 226–231. 1992.

58. **Gordon, P. B., Goldenberg, S. L., and Chan, N. H.** Solid breast lesions: diagnosis with ultrasound-guided fine needle aspiration biopsy. *Radiology* 189: 573–580, 1993.

59. **Fisher, B., Redmond, C., Poisson, R., et al.** Eight year results of a randomized clinical trial comparing total mastectomy and lumpectomy with or without irradiation in the treatment of breast cancer. *N. Engl. J. Med.* 320: 822, 1989.

60. **Veronesi, U., Salvadori, B., Luini, A., et al.** Conservative treatment of early breast cancer. *Ann. Surg.* 211: 250, 1990.

61. **Lynch, H. T., Watson, P., Conway, T., et al.** DNA screening for breast/ovarian cancer susceptibility based on linked markers. *Arch. Intern. Med.* 153: 1979–1987, 1993.

62. **Mulvihill, J. J., Safyer, A. W., and Bening, J. K.** Prevention in familial breast cancer. Counselling and prophylactic mastectomy. *Preventive Med.* 11: 500–511, 1982.

63. **Nayfield, S. G., Karp, J. E., Ford, J. E., et al.** Potential role of tamoxifen in prevention breast cancer. *J. Natl. Cancer Inst.* 32: 1450–1459, 1991.

64. **Van Nagell, J. R., DePriest, P. D., Gallion, H. H., et al.** Ovarian cancer screening. *Cancer* 71: 1523–1528, 1993.

65. **Muto, M. G., Cramer, D. W., and Brown, D. L., et al.** Screening for ovarian cancer: the preliminary experience of a familial ovarian cancer center. *Gynecol. Oncol.* 49: 112, 1993.

66. **Bourne, T. H., Campbell, S., Reynolds, K. M., et al.** Screening for early familial ovarian cancer with transvaginal ultrasonography and colour blood flow imaging. *Br. Med. J.* 306: 1025–1029, 1993.

67. **Chen, K. T. K., Schooler, J. L., and Flam, M. S.** Peritoneal carcinomatosis after prophylactic oophorectomy in familial ovarian cancer syndrome. *Obstet. Gynecol.* 66(Suppl): 935–945, 1985.

68. **Tobacman, J. K., Tucker, M. A., Kase, R., et al.** Intra-abdominal carcinomatosis after prophylactic oophorectomy in ovarian cancer prone families. *Lancet* 2: 795–797, 1982.

69. **Steinberg, K. K., Thacker, S. B., Smith, S. J., et al.** A meta-analysis of the effect of estrogen replacement therapy on the risk of breast cancer. *JAMA* 265: 1985–90, 1991.

70. **Blair, Valerie, Steinberg, Karen K.** Breast Cancer and Estrogen Therapy (Letter). *J. Am. Med. Assoc.* 13: 1001, 1994.

71. **Cobleigh, M. A., Berris, R. F., Bush, T., et al.** Estrogen replacement therapy in breast cancer survivors. A time for change. Breast Cancer Committees of the Easter Cooperative Oncology Group. *J. Am. Med. Assoc.* 272: 540–5, 1994.

72. **Vasen, H. F., Mecklin, J.-P., Watson, P., et al.** Surveillance in hereditary nonpolyposis colorectal cancer: an international cooperative study of 165 families. *Dis. Colon Rect.* 36: 1–4, 1993.

73. **Bronner, C. E., Baker, S. M., Morrison, P. T., et al.** Mutation in the DNA mismatch

repair gene homologue hMLH1 is associated with hereditary non-polyposis colon cancer. *Nature* 368 (6468: 258–61, 1994.

74. **Papadopoulos, N., Nicolaides, N. C., Wei, Y. F., et al.** Mutation of a mutL homolog in hereditary color cancer [see comments]. *Science* 263: 1625–9, 1994.
75. **Fishel, R., Lescoe, M. K., Rao, M. R., et al.** The human mutator gene homolog MSH2 and its association with hereditary nonpolyposis colon cancer. *Cell* 75: 1027–38, 1993.
76. **Leach F. S., Nicolaides, N. C., Papadopoulos, N., et al.** Mutations of a MutS homolog MSH2 and its association with hereditary nonpolyposis colon cancer. *Cell* 75: 1215–1225, 1993.
77. **Nystrom-Lahti, M., Parsons, R., Sistonen, P., et al.** Mismatch repair genes on chromosomes 2p and 3p account for a major share of hereditary nonpolyposis colorectal cancer. *Am. J. Hum. Genet.* 1994. (in press)
78. **Nicolaides, N. C., Papadopoulos, N., Wei, Y-F, et al.** Mutations of two PMS homologues in hereditary nonpolyposis colorectal cancer. *Nature* 371: 75–80, 1994.
79. **Lynch, H. T., Harris, R. E., Lynch, P. M., et al.** Role of heredity in multiple primary cancer. *Cancer* 40: 1949–1854, 1977.
80. **Lynch, H. T., Smyrk, T. C., Watson, P., et al.** Genetics, natural history, tumor spectrum and pathology of hereditary nonpolyposis colorectal cancer. An updated review. *Gastroenterology* 104: 1535–1549, 1993.
81. **Mecklin, J. P. and Harvinen, H. H.** Clinical features of colorectal carcinoma in cancer family syndrome. *Dis. Colon Rect.* 29: 160–164, 1986.
82. **Lynch, P. and Winn, R. J.** Clinical management of hereditary nonpolyposis colon cancer. *Hematol. Oncol. Clin. North Am.* 3(1): 75–86.
83. **Mecklin, J.-P. and Harvinen, H.** Treatment and follow-up strategies in hereditary nonpolyposis colorectal cancer. *Dis. Colon Rect.* 36: 927–929, 1993.
84. **Watson, P., Vasen, H. F., Mecklin, J. P., Jarvinen, H., and Lynch, H. T.** The risk of endometrial cancer in hereditary nonpolyposis colorectal cancer. *Am. J. Med.* 96(6): 516–20, 1994.
85. **Watson, P.** Report of the fifth meeting of the ICG-HNPCC. p1, 1993.
86. **Watson, P. and Lynch, H. T.** Extracolonic cancer in hereditary nonpolyposis colorectal cancer. *Cancer* 71: 677–685, 1993.
87. **Vasen, H. F. A., Offeraus, G. J., den Hartog-Jager, F. C., et al.** The tumor spectrum in hereditary nonpolyposis colorectal cancer. A study of 24 kindreds in the Netherlands. *Int. J. Cancer* 46: 31–34, 1990.
88. **Mecklin, J.-P. and Jarvinen, H. J.** Tumor spectrum in cancer family syndrome (Hereditary Nonpolyposis Colorectal Cancer). *Cancer* 68: 1109–1112, 1991.
89. **Bulow, S., Burn, J., Neale, K., Northover, J., and Vasen, H.** The establishment of a polyposis register. *Int. J. Colorectal Dis.* 8(1): 34–8, 1993.
90. **Northover, J. M.** Activities of the Leeds Castle Polyposis Group. *Semin. Surg. Oncol.* 3(2): 118–9, 1987.
91. **Vasen, H. F., Griffioen, G., Offerhaus, G. J., et al.** The value of screening and central registration of families with familial adenomatous polyposis. A study of 82 families in The Netherlands. *Dis. Colon Rect.* 33(3): 227–30, 1990.
92. **Gayther, S.l A., Wells, D., SenGupta, S. B., et al.** Regionally clustered APC mutations are associated with a severe phenotype and occur at a high frequency in new mutation cases of adenomatous polyposis coli. *Hum. Mol. Genet.* 3(1): 53–6, 1994.
93. **Powell, S. M., Petersen, G. M., Krush, A. J., et al.** Molecular diagnosis of familial adenomatous polyposis. *N. Engl. J. Med.* 329(27): 1982–7, 1993.
94. **Eckert, W. A., Jung, C., and Wolff, G.** Presymptomatic diagnosis in families with adenomatous polyposis using highly polymorphic dinucleotide CA repeat markers flanking the APC gene. *J. Med. Genet.* 31(6): 442–7, 1994.
95. **Herrera, L., O'Riordan, B. G., and Cambronero, E.** Familial adenomatous polyposis.

Surg. Oncol. Clin. North Am. 3(3): 419–434, 1994.

96. **Burt, R. W.** Polyposis syndromes. *Textbook of Gastroenterology.* Yamada T. Ed. Lippincott, New York, 1674–1696, 1991.

97. **Lynch, H. T., Fitzgibbons, R., Jr., Chong, S., et al.** Use of doxorubicin and dacarbazine for the management of unresectable intra-abdominal desmoid tumors in Gardner"s syndrome. *Dis. Colon Rect.* 37: 260–7, 1994.

98. **Patel, S. R., Evans, H. L., and Benjamin, R. S.** Combination chemotherapy in adult desmoid tumors. *Cancer* 72: 3244–7, 1993.

99. **Acker, J. C., Bossen, E. H., and Halperin, E. C.,** The management of desmoid tumors. *Int. J. Radiat. Oncol. Biol. Phys.* 26: 851–8, 1993.

100. **Seiter, K. and Kemeny, N.** Successful treatment of a desmoid tumor with doxorubicin. *Cancer* 71: 2242–4, 1993.

101. **de Mestier, P.** Cancer thyroidien et polypose recto-colique familiale. *Chirurgie* 116(6-7): 514–6, 1990.

102. **Herrera, L., Carrel, A., Rao, U., et al.** Familial adenomatous polyposis in association with thyroiditis. Report of two cases. *Dis. Colon Rect.* 32: 893–6, 1989.

103. **Creaver, P. J., Pendyala, N., Petrelli, et al.** Phase I study of difluoromethylornithine (DFMO) as a chemopreventive agent (CPA). *Proc. Am. Soc. Clin. Oncol.* 11: 144, 1992.

104. **Waddell, W. R.** The effect of sulindac on colon polyps: circumvention of a transformed phenotype — a hypothesis. *J. Surg. Oncol.* 55: 52–5, 1994.

105. **Herrera, L.** Editorial comments on Waddel WR.: the effect of sulindac on colon polyps. Circumvention of a transformed phenotype. A hypothesis. *J. Surg. Oncol.* 55: 55, 1994.

106. **Labayle, D., Fischer, D., Vielh, P., et al.** Sulindac causes regression of rectal polyps in familial adenomatous polyposis. *Gastroenterology* 101: 635–9, 1991.

107. **Lotfi, A. M., Dozois, R. R., Gordon, H., et al.** Mesenteric fibromatosis complicating familial adenomatous polyposis: predisposing factors and results of treatment. *Int. J. Colorectal Dis.* 4: 30–6, 1989.

108. **Welling, D. R. and Dozois, R. R.** The ileal pouch-anal anastomosis: surgical technique and current clinical results. *Ann. Acad. Med. Singapore* 16: 529–31, 1987.

109. **Dozois, R. R.** Restorative proctocolectomy and ileal reservoir. *Mayo Clin. Proc.* 61(4): 283–6, 1986.

110. **Sandborn, W. J., Tremaine, W. J., Batts, K. P., et al.** Pouchitis after ileal pouch-anal anastomosis: a Pouchitis Disease Activity Index. *Mayo Clin. Proc.* 69: 409–15, 1994.

Chapter 9

GENETIC COUNSELING AND CANCER

Hansjakob Müller

CONTENTS

I. INTRODUCTION

Science is coming closer to defining germ-line mutations involved in the etiology of late onset disorders such as various types of cancer.[1,2] A growing number of germ-line mutations can be identified before clinical symptoms occur. Due to this progress in predictive or presymptomatic testing through more frequent monitoring, cancers can be identified at the earliest stages of development when treatability is best. Therefore, genetic counseling of cancer patients and their relatives is becoming an important task in oncology. It should be offered to all persons at an increased cancer risk, irrespective of whether it is suggested by the medical profession or by the counselee.

Genetic counseling is a communication process which deals with the human problems associated with the occurrence, or risk of occurrence, of a genetic disorder.[3] It involves diagnosis, risk assessment, explanations, and the choice

0-8493-4782-3/96/$0.00+$.50
© 1996 by CRC Press Inc.

of options, and may have a bearing on the health of familiy members other than the individual being counseled.[4,5]

In the context of cancer, genetic counseling may be desirable in one of the following three settings:[6] (1) at the time of diagnosis to address questions of causation (etiology); (2) at the time of therapy, to address issues of reproduction and possible teratogenicity; (3) after successful treatment, to address the possibility of recurrence, risks in relatives, and reproductive issues. This review concentrates on issues of genetic counseling related to testing for cancer predispositions.

II. THE PROCESS OF GENETIC COUNSELING

There is no single, perfect technique of genetic counseling. Its goals are so comprehensive that a single approach can hardly encompass the varied needs of people who seek help. This leads to considerable variability in genetic counseling as provided in the different medical settings and also envisioned by the community of medical geneticists. The main considerations[7] involved in the process of genetic counseling and aspects specific to cancer are listed in Table 1.

An **accurate diagnosis** of the underlying susceptibility using all modern medical modalities is the cornerstone of genetic counseling because most

TABLE 1
Genetic Counseling — Aspects Specific to Cancer

Element of genetic counseling	Aspects specific to cancer
Accurate diagnosis of the predisposition (susceptibility)	• Heterogeneity
	• Reduced life expectancy of patients (relatives)
	• Late manifestation of the disease
	• Variable expressivity and penetrance of the trait
	• New germ-line mutations
Risk determination (recurrence)	• Difficult to assess with conventional methods if gene tracking not possible
Communication of genetic and medical facts	• Many medical professionals involved
	• Acceptance of information and advice by both patients and physicians
Evaluation of possible options and alternatives	• Associated neoplasms (which cancer to screen for and how often?)
Follow-up and continuing support of the counselee and his/her family members	• Change of family doctor and of family relationship

cancers seem to have multiple causes. A wrong diagnosis may have devastating consequences. A precise genetic diagnosis can be more easily achieved in rare disorders such as the hamartomatous syndromes (neurofibromatosis 1, von Hippel-Lindau syndrome, tuberous sclerosis) which show unequivocal clinical symptoms. It is more difficult to reliably determine a predisposition to the more common cancers. Recently, however, individual genes predisposing to colorectal and breast cancer have been identified. The genes (*hMSH2* and *hMLH1*, *PMS1* and *PMS2*) for colorectal cancer are responsible for the DNA mismatch repair system[8] while the functions of *BRCA1* and *BRCA2*, which lead, if mutated, to mammary carcinoma,[9] are currently being studied. The p53 gene on chromosome 17p is mutated in several families with the Li-Fraumeni syndrome characterized by the familial occurrence of breast cancer of early onset, soft-tissue sarcoma in childhood, brain tumor, osteosarcoma, leukemia, and adrenocortical carcinoma.[10] In the search to define the nature and extent of the genetic heterogeneity underlying inherited susceptibilities to common cancers, studies based on families referred for counseling will be of considerable importance.

A thoroughly compiled family history of cancer is potentially the most beneficial component of the patient's work-up and can, in particular, give clues for the presence of a susceptibility to breast or colorectal cancer. The family history often gives important information on who should be genetically tested and what test should be used. However, the family cancer history still is often the most neglected portion of the patient's medical evaluation. The pedigree analysis gives only limited information when the family is small or when little or no information on affected relatives is available. Many familial cancers develop only late in adult life, so that relatives at risk may still be healthy at the time of compiling the family history. Furthermore, with regard to the familial occurrence of common cancers such as breast cancer, aggregation of sporadic forms due only to somatic mutations may be found in certain families.

The result of pedigree analysis is also subject to methodological errors.[11,12] In general, women are better informed about their families and more information is usually available concerning relatives on the maternal rather than on the paternal side. The more distant the relatives, the lower is the percentage of persons reported to have cancer. When anamnesis is incomplete, additional investigations are indicated: medical records or autopsy reports must be evaluated. The willingness to cooperate in pedigree analysis has shown itself to be a good indicator of receptivity to subsequent counseling.

Molecular genetic tests are allowing more "cancer" genes inherited through the germ-line to be detected in an individual before clinical symptoms occur. However, genetic tests are seldom perfect predictors of clinical risk. Allelic and genetic diversity occurs in most genetic disorders. The detection of an alteration can only indicate susceptibility and cannot predict with certainty the occurrence of a given cancer. Thus, it becomes important to distinguish between analytic sensitivity (the ability of a test to detect the various mutations it was designed to detect) and clinical sensitivity (the ability of the test to detect all patients who will develop or who have the disease). In cases of incomplete penetrance the specific mutation may be a necessary but not sufficient condition for the disease to become manifest. It has to be kept in mind that genetic test information on predispositions to cancer has a potential to falsely label persons as being at risk for the disease even though they are gene carriers.

Reliable assessment of the **genetic risk** in relatives of a patient with a given cancer may be difficult. There are several ways of determing this risk in a given family: (1) by determination of the empirical risk, (2) by calculation of the so-called analytical risk, (3) by indirect DNA-diagnostic procedures or (4) by direct DNA-diagnostic procedures. The empirical risk is determined by observing the incidence of neoplasms in relatives of persons with the same or an associated malignancy. Murphy and Chase[3] developed an alternative method of genetic risk assessment using a genetic model for risk evaluation in a given family. DNA-based tests permit the presymptomatic identification of the individual at-risk relative.[14] It became possible to search for family members who have inherited the predisposition and to offer them specific information about their risk of passing the trait on to their children.[15] Indirect DNA diagnosis relies on genetic linkage and uses DNA polymorphisms to track a specific gene within a family. In direct DNA diagnosis, a search is made for the presence or absence of a specific mutant allele at a defined locus. Neoplasms with several genetic causes limit a direct approach. Until specific genes are found for common cancers, empiric risk estimates have to be offered which can be modified by the consideration of other individual risk factors.[16] Also, predictive or presymptomatic testing and screening can only provide clues about a genetic susceptibility to cancer. The nature of the prediction will usually be probabilistic (certain degree of likelihood) and not deterministic (without doubt). Caution in the use and interpretation of the test results is indicated.

Genetic counseling is a multifaceted process that involves more than an accurate diagnosis and risk assessment. The counselee expects and deserves an accurate and reasonable answer to his other queries about the known susceptibility to a particular cancer or the implications of the result of predictive testing[17] (Table 2). In order to meet the necessity of helping the counselee and his/her family, it is necessary to identify personal goals and values so that workable decisions can be made.[18] The counselor needs didactic and psychological skill to explain complex medical, genetic, and psychological facts (see Table 3). Informative counseling is time-consuming. Often several sessions are needed in order to arrive at the goal. In the first session, the counselee may not be as receptive as in later sessions when some of the early shock and denial that accompany cancer diagnosis has abated.

Today, there is a growing possibility of using alternatives in genetic counseling such as interactive video or computer methods, thus improving the communication of information.

In the discussion with the counselee, problems may develop due to the involvement of an unusual number of professionals from various medical

TABLE 2
Range of Questions and Issues for Those Considering Genetic Testing

- What is the nature and the severity of the disorder?
- What does the future hold for health, longevity, quality of life?
- How reliable is the test?
- What does genetic information mean for me, for my children, for my entire family, for future generations?
- What medical and support services will be needed and/or will be available?
- What does the genetic information mean for future insurability, employability, personal and social stigmas, and discrimination?
- How great are the risks of the test?

TABLE 3
Genetic counseling has to be

- As understandable as possible
- As sympathetic as possible
- As accurate as possible
- As scientific as necessary

disciplines who hold different views. It is often of special importance that questions related to the pathogenesis of a given cancer are evaluated in joint consultation and are not communicated among the various specialists using the patient as a "go-between". If several professionals are involved in the precounseling diagnostic and genetic work-up, it is advisable to hold conferences with them to make sure that no facet has been overlooked and that there is no misunderstanding between the experts.

The possible **options** for dealing with the genetic burden are evaluated in several contributions in this volume. Identification of most persons at risk for certain cancers suggests that more frequent monitoring may identify the earliest manifestations of a newly developing neoplasm.[7] The ultimate goals of counseling and monitoring are the treatment, cure, and possible prevention of genetic disease, but effective interventions lag behind the ability to detect cancer or increased susceptibilities to cancer.

To ensure that counseling achieves its goals, it has to be evaluated by formal or informal methods. This can be an oral short-answer quiz to estimate the retention of information, or a more formal approach which also permits comparison between counselors or counseling techniques. A long-term follow-up, as well as continuing support for the counselee and his/her relatives, is very important in order to avoid unnecessary anxieties as well as for the prevention of incurable cancer by regular screening and early diagnosis.

Sporadic cancers of primarily unkown etiology pose special problems for genetic counseling. The etiology of sporadic cancer includes new germ-line mutations, autosomal recessive inheritance, uniparental disomy, germinal mosaicism in one parent, or other influences.

III. WHO NEEDS GENETIC COUNSELING FOR CANCER?

There are many features (see Table 4) that suggest that a person has cancer due to a genetic susceptibility. Some factors were found only by case series, and others were identified by analytic, epidemiologic, and by molecular genetic studies.[6] Genetic counseling should be offered to all persons at an increased cancer risk independent of whether it is suggested by the medical profession or by the counselee.

In the ninth edition of *Mendelian Inheritance in Man*, McKusick[19] lists 2636 definite single-gene traits and 2281 others with suggestive but inconclusive evidence of Mendelian inheritance behavior. Of the 4917 traits, 338 conditions (in addition to 56 protoncogenes) have neoplasia as the sole feature, a frequent concomitant, or a rare complication.[20,21]

IV. BASIC TENETS OF GENETIC COUNSELING

The basic tenets of genetic counseling are listed in Table 5. The presentation and discussion of the medical and genetic facts have to be made in simple nontechnical language. Illustrative material may be of help in the explanation of the pathophysiological and genetic features of a cancer susceptibility. The counselor must promote interaction with the counselee. The educational level of the counselee correlates with the amount of information retained: the higher the education, the better the counselee can assimilate complicated concepts. However, few persons understand probability theories or are familiar with the statistical principles of odds or risks of occurrence.[22]

Nondirectiveness[23] should always be a basic principle of reproductive planning and decisions. Information, concepts, and options must be presented in a way so balanced as not to influence the counselee in a particular fashion. Since risk perceptions vary among individuals and also among counselors, there is no single correct way of presenting or interpreting genetic risk information. Ethical and cultural sensitivity is particularly important in view of cultural differences between the client and the health care professional. Obviously, the counselor can never be completely neutral and the counselee often wants to learn his personal view.

Voluntariness should be the cornerstone of any presymptomatic testing program for cancer. The decision to carry out, continue, or stop the investigation rests exclusively with the counselee, who will also decide whether and to what extent they wish to be informed and to draw conclusions from, the test

TABLE 4
Who Needs Genetic Counseling?

A predisposition to cancer has to be considered when neoplasms occur:
- In more than two generations
- In several foci within one organ
- In both of paired organs
- In siblings
- At an unsual age for the tumor type
- In association with certain other cancers
- In defined genetic disorders/birth defects

TABLE 5
Basic Tenets of Genetic Counseling

- Nondirectiveness
- Recognition of social and cultural differences
- Voluntariness/Informed consent
- Confidentiality

results. Informed consent has been accepted as an essential component of every doctor-patient relationship. Minors capable of judgment and legally incapacitated persons under guardianship have their own right of decision. In the case of persons incapable of judgment, the consent of their legal representative is required.

For results obtained in the course of genetic investigation, the same rules governing professional medical secrecy and data protection apply as for other medical data. It is the right and responsibility of the individual to determine who shall have access to medical information, particularly the results of presymptomatic testing for cancer. However, if there is a possible medical need for informing an individual's blood relative, steps should be taken to provide them with the relevant genetic data, but only with the consent of the person tested .

V. PSYCHOLOGICAL AND ETHICAL ASPECTS IN GENETIC COUNSELING OF CANCER

The problems encountered in genetic counseling for cancer differ partly from those involved in noncancerous diseases.[24] The counselee is frequently an adult who has already had the desired number of children. He may hold himself responsible for the increased cancer risk to his progeny and feel guilty for it. Some situations have an almost overwhelming psychological impact, requiring psychotherapeutic interaction before, during, or after genetic counseling. Profound emotional responses may be shown by the entire family, including spouses, once the risk to other family members becomes known. Even favorable news and the reassurance of not being a carrier of a susceptibility can affect people's concepts of themselves and their families, and may lead to what is called "survivor guilt".[25]

Genetic counseling includes both empathetic and emotional support as a part of the entire process. The counselee frequently needs to be encouraged to express his feelings and conflicts. The motivation and the emotional state of the counselee are probably the most important factors for the effectiveness of the communication process. A counselee who is hostile, seriously depressed, or anxious is likely to take in information either inaccurately or incompletely. Some experienced counselors, therefore, think that the psychotherapeutic aspect of counseling is much more important than the communication of medical and genetic facts.[26] The benefits of the various presymptomatic interventions must be weighed against potential anxiety, stigmatization, and other possible harm to individuals who are informed that they are at increased risk of developing cancer. The counselor acts as a resource in dealing with the sadness, loss, anger, guilt, or anxiety that genetic information can bring.

In our own study, with the goal of learning more about the attitudes of patients with breast and colorectal cancer as well as that of their relatives at risk, with respect to genetic counseling in general and active genetic counseling in particular, it was found that only a few probands expressed reservations concerning the practice of contacting and informing relatives of patients.[27]

If the diagnostic work-up indicates that the occurrence of cancer is not related to a significant genetic element, this fact has to be explained clearly to the counselee in order to avoid a lifelong fear of carrying a cancer predisposition.

The setting in which a counseling session occurs may influence the quality and outcome of communication. In some families, it proves fruitful to talk to all persons at risk of cancer, while in others it is preferable to hold the discussion with each person separately.

Research is needed on the psychological implications of genetic counseling and presymptomatic testing in both adults and children.

VI. POPULATION SCREENING

The identification of mutated genes predisposing to cancer makes population-based genetic screening a potential part of routine health care. However, population screening for predispositions to cancer should only be considered for preventable or treatable conditions at high frequency.[28] The sole goal of reducing the incidence of genetic conditions is not acceptable, since this aim alone is explicitly eugenic.[17] Screening programs cannot fulfill their aims unless the persons to be tested are aware of the purpose of the test, the disease or predisposition it is intended to detect, its availability, its benefits to individuals, and its limitations. Genetic counseling is the context for helping people address such issues. The voluntary nature of participation in the presymptomatic testing and the right not to be informed of the result must also be guaranteed for all screening examinations.

Direct DNA testing for the single gene defects such as those predisposing to breast or colorectal cancer should only be provided in specialized genetic centers familiar with genetic counseling and the psychosocial aspects of predictive testing. Neither family physicians nor clinicians are sufficiently prepared to deal with the complexities of counseling for late-onset disorders.

VII. CONCLUSION

The family physician is the key person in the management of the counselee and in the interaction between specialized clinicians, medical geneticists, laboratory scientists, and many others. He should, therefore, familiarize himself with modern molecular genetics, as this discipline has an increasingly important place in the diagnosis, treatment, and prevention of cancer. If he is unable to meet the requirement for proper genetic counseling with the expertise and depth that may be required he should seek advice from trained medical geneticists or refer his patient to such colleagues. The complexities of the underlying mechanisms involved in determining and establishing susceptibility, in sorting out potential environmental influences, and, finally, in devising a strategy for counseling will present challenges in the future.

ACKNOWLEGMENT

Our own results on familial cancer were collected with the support of the Swiss National Fund (Grants 32-30007.90 and 32-32556.91).

REFERENCES

1. **Müller, H.-J.,** Dominant inheritance of human cancer. *Anticancer Res.*, 10, 505–512, 1990.
2. **Müller, H.-J.,** Recessively inherited deficiencies predisposing to cancer, *Anticancer Res.*, 10, 513–518, 1990.
3. **Ad hoc Committee on Genetic Counseling,** Report to the American Society of Human Genetics, *Am. J. Hum. Genet.*, 27, 240–242, 1975.
4. **Fraser, F. C.,** Genetic counseling, *Am. J. Hum. Genet.*, 26, 638–659, 1974.
5. **Emery, A. E.,** Genetic counseling, *Br. Med. J.*, 3, 219, 1975.
6. **Mulvihill, J. J.,** Genetic counseling of the cancer patients, in *Cancer: Principles and Practice of Medical Oncology,* DeVita, V. T., Jr, Hellman, S., Rosenberg, S. A., 4th ed. 1993, chap. 65.
7. **Müller, H.-J., Scott, R., Weber, W., and Meier, R.,** Colorectal cancer: lessons for genetic counselling and care for families, *Clin. Genet.*, 46, 106–114, 1994.
8. **Jiricny, J.,** Colon cancer and DNA repair: have mismatches met their match?, *TIG*, 10,

164–168, 1994.

9. **Wooster, R. and Stratton, M. R.,** Breast cancer susceptibility: a complex diesease unravels. *TIG,* 11, 3-5, 1995.

10. **Malkin, D.,** p53 and the Li-Fraumeni syndrome, *Cancer Genet. Cytogenet.,* 66, 83–92, 1993.

11. **Müller, H.-J.,** Familial cancer in Basel: some aspects, in Müller, H.-J. and Weber, W., Eds., *Familial Cancer,* S. Karger, Basel, 1985, 1–5.

12. **Bondy, M. L., Strom, S. S., Colopy, M. W., Brown, B. W., and Strong, L. C.,** Accuracy of family history of cancer obtained through interviews with relatives of patients with childhood sarcoma, *J. Clin. Epidemiol.,* 47, 89–96, 1994.

13. **Murphy, E. A. and Chase, G. A.,** *Principles of genetic counselling,* Year Book, 1975.

14. **Müller. Hj. and Scott, R.,** Hereditary conditions in which loss of heterozygosity may be important, *Mutat. Res.,* 284, 15–24, 1992.

15. **Müller, Hj.,** Patients without disease? Benefits and risks of presymptomatic testing, *Schweiz. Rundsch. Med.,* 82, 45–49, 1993.

16. **Geil, M. H., Brinton, L. A., Byar, D. P., et al.,** Projecting individualized probabilities on developing breast cancer for white females who are being examined annually, *JNCI,* 81, 1879–1886, 1989.

17. **Andrews, L. B., Fullarton, J. E., Holtzman, N. A., and Motulsky, A. G., Eds.,** *Assessing Genetic Risks,* National Academy Press, Washington, D. C., 1994.

18. **Erbe, R. W.,** Genetic counseling, in *Textbook of Internal Medicine,* Kelley, W. N., et al., Eds., J. B. Lippincott, Philadelphia, 1988, 2343–2349.

19. **McKusick, V. A.,** *Mendelian Inheritance in Man,* 9th ed., Johns Hopkins University Press, Baltimore, 1990.

20. **Müller, H.-J. and Scott, R.,** How common is hereditary cancer? *Ann. Med.,* 26, 173–175, 1994.

21. **Hodgson, S. V. and Maher, E. R.,** *A Practical Guide to Human Cancer Genetics,* Cambridge University Press, Cambridge, 1993.

22. **Lolouel, J. M.,** Probability calculations in pedigrees under complex modes of inheritance, *Hum. Hered.,* 30, 320–323, 1980.

23. **Kessler, S.,** Psychological aspects of genetic counseling. VII. Thoughts on directiveness, *J. Clin. Counseling,* 1, 9–17, 1992.

24. **Lynch, H. T., Lynch, P. M., and Lynch, J. F.,** in *Genetic Counseling,* Kessler, S., Ed., Academic Press, New York, 1979, 221–241.

25. **Wexler, N.,** The Tiresias complex: Huntington's disease as a paradigm of testing for late-onset disorders, *FASEB J.,* 6, 2820–2925, 1992.

26. **Money, J.,** Counseling in genetics and applied behavior genetics, in *Developmental Human Behavior Genetic,* Schaie, K. W., Anderson, V. E., McClearn, G. E., and Money, J., Eds., Lexington Books, Lexington, 1975.

27. **Ruefli, C. and Müller, H.-J.,** Genetische Beratung bei familiären Kolon- und Mammakarzinom: wie stellen sich Betroffene dazu? *Schweiz. Krebs—Bull., 2,* 10–13, 1989.

28. **Hampton, M. L., Anderson, J., Lavizzo, B. S., and Bergman, A. B.,** Sickle cell "nondisease". A potentially serious public health problem, *Am. J. Dis. Child.,* 128, 58–61, 1974.

Chapter 10

SCREENING FOR FAMILIAL CANCER

Lennart Iselius and Nils Wilking

CONTENTS

I. INTRODUCTION

There are several ways to reduce mortality in cancer. One can use prevention, screening, and treatment. Screening has the potential to be the most powerful tool to achieve reduced mortality in cancer. The criteria for screening are as follows:

The disease should be common and be a major health problem.
The disease should have a silent early stage.

There should be an adequate method for diagnosing the disease.

The disease should also be possible to treat in such a way that the prognosis can be improved.

However, there are several problems with screening that possibly will reduce its potential. With screening, the prognosis for some patients will be improved but this is not true for all patients. The patients who benefit from screening are those who otherwise may have developed advanced disease and would have died from the malignancy. With screening one may also detect cancer at an earlier stage than without screening. For some patients this will mean that major surgery is not necessary; for example, a quadrantectomy can be preformed instead of a modified radical mastectomy in women with breast cancer. Also, those patients who are negative at the screening may benefit from the reassurance that they are not likely to have cancer at the screened site. There may also be financial benefits for society, especially if earlier detection leads to less radical and less costly treatment.

The disadvantages of screening are the following. Earlier detection may lead to a longer period of morbidity for patients where the screening detection does not alter the course of the disease. One may also overtreat certain premalignant lesions. Patients may also get false reassurance from the screening process if they belong to the false negative screening group. In these patients, symptoms and sites of malignant disease may be recognized later because of the false reassurance from the screening process. Cases who have a false positive screening test may also undergo a series of different unnecessary investigations before they are diagnosed as not having the disease for which they have been screened. The screening test itself, like repeated radiation, may also induce morbidity.

There are several obstacles that may interfere with the success of screening in cancer control. Many cancers have an unfavorable natural history, and some may be difficult to screen; in other conditions, the compliance may be poor, especially for those at a high risk of developing the disease. For many cancers, a valid and effective screening test is not yet available. Also, some screening situations are presently too costly and have too high a morbidity to be accepted by the general public. It is important to remember, when introducing a screening program, that the disease should be an important health concern. One should be able to detect the disease in a preclinical phase and the natural history of lesions identified by screening should be known. There should be an effective treatment for the disease or its preclinical phase and the screening test should be acceptable, safe, and economical.

It is therefore very important to evaluate all screening programs thoroughly. The test used for the screening should have an adequate sensitivity (i.e., detect those who have the disease), and a high specificity (i.e., proportion of those free of disease who test negative). The screening process should also be acceptable for those who are invited to be screened. All screening programs ought to be evaluated in controlled randomized trials. Thus one may detect several of the biases that are linked to the screening process: one bias being lead-time, the time by which diagnosis is advanced by screening; and another the length bias, the tendency of screening to detect cases of disease with a more prolonged natural history and a better prognosis than normal. A screening program may also introduce a selection bias, i.e., recruit patients who are more willing and may have a different risk of the disease compared to the general population. A screening program may also introduce an overdiagnosis bias, with a tendency of the screening to bring into light disease lesions that may never have been diagnosed as a true malignancy during the patient's lifetime. Thus, the only way to design a randomized study is to use mortality in the population screened for a different disease so that one can avoid other different biases like lead-time, length, and overdiagnosis. It is also crucial that one does not employ screening in diseases where there is not an adequate set-up for diagnosis and treatment of the disease. It is of no meaning to diagnose a disease which cannot be treated.

Familial cancer represents a specific problem with respect to screening. Even though only a small fraction of cancer is inherited in a Mendelian fashion, over 200 single gene disorders have been linked to neoplasia. Hereditary neoplasms tend to occur earlier in life than other cancers of the same anatomic type. Also, they are often multifocal in origin. Some of the common neoplasms, such as breast cancer and colon cancer, show a small familial increased risk in the order of two to three. However, among subgroups of patients, one may find bilateral or multifocal disease and the risk may be as high as 20- to 30-fold. Some families show a remarkable aggregation of site-specific cancers that appear consistent with autosomal dominant inheritance. Since cancer is a common disease, it is sometimes difficult to know whether an aggregation of cases within a family is simply due to chance. There are also aggregations within families involving multiple cancer syndromes. For example, in Li-Fraumeni syndrome one will find soft tissue and bone sarcomas, breast carcinomas, brain tumors, leukemia, and adrenocortical neoplasms. It has been shown that in this syndrome the family has a germ-line mutation of p53, a tumor suppressor gene on chromosome 17p13 that often occurs as somatic mutations in a number of human cancers.[1] A multidisciplinary approach to familial cancer, ranging from clinical observations and epidemiology to molecular biology, might identify carcinogenic mechanisms and may have consequences in cancer prevention.

Before the decision is made to screen for hereditary cancer in a family the following questions must be addressed.

What is the evidence in the family for hereditary cancer? — To be able to answer this question it is mandatory that a proper family history is taken. At a minimum, the status of all first- and second-degree relatives should be asked about. All too often, a patient presents with an incurable cancer and when asked about the family history it is obvious that one is dealing with a hereditary cancer. Such an unnecessary situation may in many instances be prevented if physicians take their time to take the family history and start to screen for cancer in the family. The importance of obtaining medical notes for relatives reported to have had cancer cannot be overestimated. Often, the diagnosis reported by the consultand is totally in error. Even if the diagnosis is correct, useful information about age of onset, location, bilaterality, etc. should be obtained from the medical notes. During the process of taking the family history, other individuals at risk can be identified. Of course, these persons should also be informed about their risk of developing cancer. It is, however, entirely up to the consultand to decide if he or she is willing to contact the relatives and to establish contact between the relatives and the cancer family clinic. It is wise to caution the consultand about these contacts, since it is not rare that some family members will be very unwilling to discuss these matters. They might even be unwilling to let their close relatives at risk be approached by the consultand. The consultand should be very tactful under these circumstances. The physician should never contact the consultand's relatives without the consultand having contacted them first and obtained permission.

What is the risk for the consultand to develop a cancer? — Based on the family history and the clinical characteristics of the cancer cases in the family, a reasonable estimate of the risk in the consultand's family for hereditary cancer can be made. The risk for the consultand can in some cases be calculated using information about the mode of inheritance for the disease, age-specific penetrances, and position in the pedigree. However, in many cases a clear diagnosis of hereditary cancer cannot be made. Most families are small and the presence of several cancers due to chance in the family cannot be ruled out. In such cases empirical risk figures may be used. They are usually based on the number of affected close relatives and cannot easily be used in more complicated pedigrees.

At what risk level should screening be entertained? — No general answers can be given to this question. The choice to screen must be made together with the consultand, taking all relevant information into account. It is not only the actual risk in percent that is important, but also the hazards of screening (e.g., perforation at colonoscopy), the patient's fear of developing cancer, as well as anxiety about the screening procedure.

What is the best method for screening? — Obviously, the answer depends on the type of cancer. For breast cancer, for example, mammography combined with self-examination and examination by a physician are generally recommended. For colon cancer, on the other hand, colonoscopy might not be the most obvious choice. The risk of perforation, unavailability of a skillful endoscopist, and a low-risk situation might lead to other means of screening. Some patients might rather choose a barium enema of the colon and low-risk cases might ask for testing of occult blood in the feces, although they know about the low sensitivity of this method. The best methods of screening, in the context of hereditary cancer, have not been satisfactorily evaluated.

At what age should screening start and how often should it be performed? — No good answers exist to these questions. Knowledge about the distribution of the age of onset of the hereditary form of the particular cancer present in the family can be used to decide at what age screening should start. An additional arbitrary rule is to start at least five years before the earliest age of onset in the family under study. The frequency of examination is often based on theoretical knowledge about the biological behavior of premalignant changes and cancers, the size of tumor that can be detected with the screening method, and the cost and availability of the screening method. Also, the inconveniences and hazards for the patient are important. In practice, this means that the ususal interval between examinations is 18–24 months. A long interval is more often used at an early age, with perhaps a baseline mammogram in the mid-twenties and more frequent examinations around the most likely age of onset. The age at which to stop screening must also be decided. Again, this is a compromise between biological age and health status, expected length of survival, and likely age of onset of the hereditary cancer. The decision to stop screening has, of course, to be reached after information and discussion with the consultand. In most cases, this is not a problem.

How should information about screening methods and results be given? — It is important that the consultand obtains detailed information about the actual risk of developing cancer, as well as the methods available for screening — with their advantages and disadvantages, especially with regard to the risk of the procedure. Two consultations are often necessary before one can take the decision to screen. At the first visit the family history is taken and information about the possible ways of screening are given. At the second visit the patient is asked to give more information about the family history, after having consulted relatives, and after the physician has requested medical notes on relatives from other hospitals. Also, the patient has been given time to think about the risks and benefits to make the decision to accept screening. After examination the patient is put up for a new appointment as soon as possible. It is often a nervous period waiting for the results, therefore the time between the examination and follow-up visit should be minimized. Unfortunately, when biopsies have been taken this waiting time may extend to as long as 2–3 weeks. The results of the examinations should, if at all possible, not be given on the phone. This to avoid the situation where one has to inform the patient over the phone that a cancer has been detected.

Is psychological support needed? — For many patients the presence of a family history of cancer raises thoughts about serious disease and the threat of death. The patients often seek genetic counselling just after a close relative has been diagnosed to have cancer or recently died of cancer. The visit to the cancer family clinic is therefore not only a visit to obtain exact risk figures and technical information about screening procedures;[2] this is also a visit to someone who will listen to fears for their own risk situation and their sorrow and concern about relatives with cancer. For some patients the visit to the cancer family clinic is the first step to get help in a time of crisis. Our experience is that a nurse with cancer experience who is easily available by phone is of great help in these situations[3] (see Chapter 12).

II. SCREENING METHODS BY SITE

In the following sections, the most common hereditary cancers are discussed in terms of screening. Our intention is to present the most widely used methods for screening and to give suggestions for suitable time intervals between examinations as well as the ages when screening should start.

A. REPRODUCTIVE SYSTEM
1. Breast Cancer

Breast cancer is the most common cancer in females. The strongest risk factors relate to reproductive age and family history.[45] Familial clustering of breast cancers has been reported for more than a century. Most genetic studies support the view that an autosomal dominant gene with high, but incomplete, penetrance accounts for most breast cancer families. However, it is likely that several different predisposing genes are present within most populations. Cytogenetic and loss of heterozygosity (LOH) studies in sporadic breast cancer have pointed to several candidate loci for breast cancer genes, but there is no clear consensus from these two approaches that might direct attention to any prime target region. Recent reports of tight linkage between familial breast cancer (early onset) and breast/ovarian cancer (regardless of mean age of onset) and a locus on chromosome 17q21 have led to the identification of a gene, *BRCA1*, for the breast/ovarian cancer families.[6] A much smaller proportion of familial breast cancer is accounted for by mutations in the p53 gene (17p13) and *BRCA2*, mapped to chromosome 13.[7] Not all such families fulfill the criteria for Li-Fraumeni syndrome and not all of the inherited mutations lie within exon 7 of p53. Counselling of members of breast cancer families becomes more rewarding as these genetic lesions are identified. It is essential to extend the collection of data and breast tissue as widely as possible in a pedigree to confirm linkage to a specific locus. In the course of these studies a substantial population of women at high risk of breast and other cancers will be identified.

Due to the influence of family history on the risk of breast cancer, several centers now offer counselling to members of high-risk families. It is assumed that women identified to be at high-risk can be followed closely with physical examination and regular mammography (intervals 12–18 months) in order to identify neoplasms developing at the earliest possible stage. Tables based on the age of the consultand, number of relatives, and ages of onset have been published and are helpful for obtaining risk figures in these families.[8] In breast/ovarian cancer families, screening for ovarian cancer is also mandatory (see below). The risk estimates may also become more important with the introduction of medical prevention (tamoxifen) for breast cancer, as well as a more extensive use of prophylactic mastectomy in women with a very high risk of developing breast cancer.

2. Ovarian Cancer

Ovarian cancer has the poorest prognosis of all gynecological cancers. The overall five-year survival is less than 30%. Screening methods for ovarian cancer depend of the identification of abnormalities of ovarian morphology. The use of biochemical markers are presently being developed and evaluated.[9] It is still difficult to distinguish between benign and malignant ovarian cysts. Around 10% of all ovarian cancer cases are due to autosomal dominant inheritance.[10] There are two main types of hereditary ovarian cancer: site-specific ovarian cancer and breast/ovarian cancer (see above). The site-specific form is characterized by early onset (mid-40s compared to 60 years for the nonfamilial form) and an increased risk for bilateral disease (70–80%).[11] Women with an increased risk for familial ovarian cancer should be offered annual pelvic examination, serum CA-125 determinations, and transvaginal ultrasonography screening with color Doppler imaging.[12] When the family history of ovarian cancer is striking and suggesting an autosomal dominant mode of inheritance, the women should be given the option of prophylactic oophorectomy. However, even after prophylactic oophorectomy there still is an increased risk for peritoneal carcinomatosis.

3. Uterine Cancer

Endometrial adenocarcinoma is the most common female genital malignancy. Risk factors like obesity and late menopause are well known, but the importance of genetic factors has received relatively little attention. About 15% of patients with carcinoma of the uterus have a close relative with the same disease. A proportion of these cases are associated with hereditary nonpolyposis colon cancer. However, there are also reports of site-specific hereditary endometrial carcinoma.[13] In such families, regular pelvic examinations and curettage might be of value for early diagnosis.

B. GASTROINTESTINAL SYSTEM
1. Esophagus

Genetic factors do not seem to be of importance in the etiology of squamous cell carcinoma of the esophagus,[14] except maybe in certain populations with a very high incidence of the disorder. Familial aggregation of esophageal cancer have been described in the Turkoman population in Iran[15] as well as in certain parts of China.[16]

Only in these high-risk areas might screening be of value. An interesting exception from this rule is Barrett's esophagus, associated with adeno-carcinoma, which has been described in several families. In these families, screening with endoscopy and biopsies should be performed.[17]

2. Stomach

It is not only the family of Napoleon Bonaparte that showed a high frequency of gastric cancer. A number of studies have shown that about 10–15% of cases with gastric cancer have the same disease in their family. The risk for familial disease is higher if the proband's cancer has the diffuse type of histology.[18] Cancer of the cardia also seems to be associated with familial disease to a higher extent than other localizations.[19]

Screening is of disputed value since the choice of treatment of premalignant changes like dysplasia is difficult. We screen healthy high-risk relatives in families with two cases of gastric cancer by gastroscopy, with multiple biopsies every two years. The finding of light to moderate dysplasia leads to more frequent gastroscopies, while severe dysplasia and cancer are treated by surgery.

3. Liver

Familial occurrence of hepatocellular carcinoma is rare. There are a few reports of familial aggregation in areas with a high frequency of hepatitis B infection.[20] In most cases no screening is necessary.

4. Pancreas

Familial occurrence of pancreatic cancer is generally thought to be due to chance.[21] However, a family history of pancreatic cancer is present in 6–7% of all patients with this disorder.[22] In some families the mode of inheritance seems to be autosomal dominant with incomplete penetrance.[23] There are also several rare syndromes with monogenic inheritance where pancreatic cancer is common.

In families with two or more cases of site-specific pancreatic cancer, high-risk individuals are followed with abdominal ultrasound and tumor markers (CA 19-9 and CA 50) every two years. Although tumor markers are often within normal range in the early stages of pancreatic cancer, a rise in the concentration might indicate an early cancer. The usefulness of this screening procedure remains to be shown, but our experience with these families is that family members at risk are very anxious to be examined. Many have experienced the rapid disease progress and poor prognosis in their relatives.

5. Gallbladder and Bile Ducts

Cancer of the gallbladder is the fifth most common gastrointestinal malignancy. Although common in some ethnic groups, like North American·Indians,[24] there are few reports of familial occurrence of gallbladder cancer.[25,26] Familial cancer of the bile ducts is also rare.[27] However, an association between cholangiocarcinoma and hereditary nonpolyposis colorectal carcinoma (HNPCC) has been described.[28,29] Screening with abdominal ultrasound and liver function tests might therefore be of value in some HNPCC families. Unless familial occurrence is striking, no screening is warranted in relatives of patients with cancer of the biliary tract.

6. Colon and Rectum

General population screening for colorectal cancer (CRC) has long been under debate. Recently, however, there have been studies showing that screening with colonoscopy can reduce the mortality of CRC.[30,31] It is also evident that certain high-risk groups, like patients with ulcerative colitis, could benefit from regular screening. Also, patients with a family history of colon cancer are candidates for screening. About 5–10% of all cases of colon cancer are thought to be due to monogenic inheritance.[32,33] A small proportion (about 1%) are due to conditions associated with colon polyps, especially familial adenomatous polyposis of the colon (FAP). The majority of the genetic forms of CRC consists of a mixture of syndromes inherited in an autosomal dominant fashion.[34]

Due to small family size it is often difficult to obtain secure evidence for dominant inheritance in a family. Empiric risks are therefore of great value (Table 1). Individuals with a relative risk higher than 1 in 10 or 12 should be offered screening with colonoscopy at regular intervals. We have chosen to screen every two years, but other intervals exist — with up to 5-year intervals if no adenomas are found. If adenomas are found more frequent colonoscopies are mandatory. Our experience is that two years is a reasonable interval, both for patient compliance and to minimize the risk of missing newly developed adenomas. We have had patients who in two years have developed adenomas of significant size and with severe dysplasia. It is important that the best technique available for colonoscopy is used. High-resolution imaging and indigo-carmine dyeing increase the possibilities to detect flat adenomas, which often are very difficult to distinguish from normal mucosa.

When family history and clinical findings suggest the hereditary nonpolyposis colon cancer syndrome (HNPCC),[35] most authors suggest close surveillance

TABLE 1
Risks of Colorectal Cancer in
First-Degree Relatives of
Colon Cancer Patients

Relatives affected	Risk
One relative	1 in 17
One first- and one second-degree relative	1 in 12
One relative <45 years	1 in 10
Two first-degree relatives	1 in 6
Three first-degree relatives	1 in 2

Houlston, R.S., Murday, V., Harocopos, C., Williams, C.B., and Slack, J. Screening and genetic counselling for relatives of patients with colorectal cancer in a family cancer clinic. *BMJ*, 301, 366, 1990.

with colonoscopy starting at the age of 20–25, with a screening interval, differing between clinics, of 1–3 years.[36] Some centers recommend lifelong screening while others stop at age 60–75 years. It is evident that no common policy exists and that the screening policy must depend on patient preference and availability of screening. In some HNPCC families there is an overrepresentation of extracolonic cancers, especially endometrial cancer.[37] These families are sometimes called Lynch syndrome II families and the association is called cancer family syndrome. Although a number of cancers have been thought to be overrepresented in these families, it is wise not to embark on a number of screening procedures unless the extended family history suggests that a particular cancer is common in the family.

The recent findings of linkage of HNPCC to chromosomes 2[38] and 3[39] and the further cloning of four mismatch repair genes will in the future change the care of these families. Individuals at risk will be more precisely defined and some individuals known to be carriers might opt for prophylactic colectomy.

C. URINARY SYSTEM
1. Kidney

In children, Wilm tumor has been studied extensively from a genetic point of view, and molecular genetic studies have shown the existence of at least three different genes causing this type of malignancy. In adults, several families with renal cell carcinoma (hypernephroma) have been described. Only about 1% of all cases of renal cell carcinoma are due to genetic factors. Many of the familial case are classified as von Hippel-Lindau disease, for which a detailed screening program has been published.[40] In the remaining cases we use regular ultrasound screening (annually) and CT scans (every three years).

2. Bladder

Although a small number of familial bladder cancer have been described most cases are due to environmental factors, mainly smoking, and screening is very seldom used.

3. Prostate

Screening for familial prostatic cancer suffers from the dilemma that no treatment of early cancer has been shown to be of any benefit. The effect of radical prostatectomy is still under debate. Since as many as 10% of cases with prostate cancer might be hereditary, the number of patients at risk is substantial. For high-risk cases annual palpation of the prostate together with ultrasound examination and determination of prostatic specific antigen (PSA) are used.

D. MELANOMA

The lifetime risk of developing malignant melanoma in the American Caucasian population is estimated to be 0.7% and in the black population

0.07%. It has been shown that melanoma patients have a higher sensitivity for utraviolet light. This indicates that melanoma patients have an increased sensitivity to UV-light independent of pigmentation. In xeroderma pigmentosa — a recessively inherited disease — one will see extreme sensitivity for UV-light. Sun exposure will induce ulcerations and multiple squamous cell carcinoma as well as multiple basal cell carcinoma at early age. Approximately 50% of these individuals will also develop malignant melanoma. Xeroderma pigmentosa is caused by a defect in the ability of the cell to repair DNA damage induced by UV-light. Less than 5% of the patients with malignant melanoma will belong to families with two or more relatives with the disease. First-degree relatives of patients with melanoma are at a two to eight times higher risk of developing melanoma than the general population.[41]

Through the pioneering work of Clark et al. it has been found that in these families approximately 95% of the individuals with malignant melanoma also will have dysplastic nevus syndrome[42] About 50% of the family members will also have dysplastic nevi. It has been estimated, in these dysplastic nevi families, that the lifetime risk of developing a malignant melanoma is almost 100%. In members of these families who do not have dysplastic nevus syndrom, no such increased risk has been noticed. Dysplastic nevus syndrome is inherited as an autosomal dominant trait. The syndrome may be related to genes on chromosome 9.[43]

It is important to investigate, in all cases of malignant melanoma if there are other members of the family with the disease. If at least two melanoma patients are found within the same family, one should recommend examinations of all family members with respect to melanoma and dysplastic nevus syndrome Individuals with a dysplastic nevus syndrome should be informed about sun habits and come to clinical controls two to four times yearly. Usually, it is not possible to surgically excise all nevi. However, one should recommend excision of one to three dysplastic nevi for histological verification. All dysplastic nevi should be photo documented in such a way that both colour and size can be registered. This allows the detection of various small changes in colour and size. If such changes appear, the lesion should be excised for histopathological examination.

III. CONCLUSIONS

Screening, and thereby early detection of malignant disease, is one of the most powerful tools in reducing mortality in cancer. However, there are several potential biases that may reduce the impact of screening. With respect to familial cancer it is important to define the screening method to be used, as well as the age when to start screening, and the screening interval. These variables need to be studied in a systematic way, to be able to construct optimal screening procedures for hereditary cancer.

REFERENCES

1. **Harris, C. C. and Hollstein, M.,** Clinical implications of the p53 tumor-suppressor gene. *N. Engl. J. Med.*, 329, 1318–1327, 1993.
2. **Kelly, P. T.,** Informational needs of individuals and families with hereditary cancers. *Semin. Oncol. Nursing*, 8, 288, 1992.
3. **McGuire, D. B.,** Familial cancer and the role of the nurse. *Cancer Nursing*, 2, 443, 1979.
4. **Brinton, L., Hoover, R., and Fraumeni, J. Jr.,** Reproductive factors in aetiology of breast cancer. *Br. J. Cancer*, 47, 757–762, 1983.
5. **Sattin, R., Rubin, G., and Webster, L.,** Family history and the risk of breast cancer. *JAMA*, 253, 1908–1913, 1985.
6. **Hall, J. M., Lee, M. K., Newman, B., et al.,** Linkage of early-onset familial breast cancer to chromosome 17q21. *Science*, 250, 1684, 1990.
7. **Malkin, D., Li, F. P., Strong, L. C., et al.,** Germ line p53 mutations in familial syndrome of breast cancer, sarcomas and other neoplasms. *Science*, 250, 1233, 1990.
8. **Claus, E. B., Risch, N., and Thompson, W. D.,** Autosomal dominant inheritance of early-onset breast cancer. Implications for risk prediction. *Cancer*, 73, 643, 1994.
9. **Hakama, M., Chamberlain, J., Day, N. E., et al.,** Evaluation of screening programmes for gynaecologic cancer. *Br. J. Cancer*, 52, 669–673, 1985.
10. **Houlston, R.S., Collins, A., Slack, J., Campbell, S., Collins, W. P., Whitehead, M. I., and Morton, N. E.,** Genetic epidemiology of ovarian cancer: segregation analysis. *Ann. Hum. Genet.*, 55, 291, 1991.
11. **Lynch, H. T., Watson, P., Bewtra, C., Conway, T. A., Hippee, C. R., Kaur, P., Lynch, J. F., and Ponder, B.,** Hereditary ovarian cancer. *Cancer*, 67, 1460, 1991.
12. **Lynch, H. T.,** Editorial: Genetic risks in ovarian cancer. *Gynecol. Oncol.*, 46, 1, 1992.
13. **Sandles, L. G., Shulman, L. P., Elias, S., Photopulos, G. J., Smiley, L. M., Posten, W. M., and Simpson, J. L.,** Endometrial adenocarcinoma: Genetic analysis suggesting heritable site-specific uterine cancer. *Gynecol. Oncol.*, 47, 161, 1992.
14. **Mosbech, J. and Videbaek, A.,** On the aetiology of oesophageal carcinoma. *J. Natl. Cancer Inst.*, 15, 1665, 1955.
15. **Ghadirian, P.,** Familial history of esophageal cancer. *Cancer*, 56, 2112, 1985.
16. **Hu, N., Dawsey, S. M., Wu, M., Bonney, G. E., He, L. J., Han, X., Fu, M., and Taylor, P. R.,** Familial aggregation of Oesophageal cancer in Yangcheng County, Shanxi Province, China. *Int. J. Epidemiol.*, 21, 877, 1992.
17. **Jochem, V. J., Fuerst, P. A., and Fromkes, J. J.,** Familial Barrett´s esophagus associated with adenocarcinoma. *Gastroenterology*, 102, 1400, 1992.
18. **Lehtola, J.,** Family study of gastric carcinoma; with special reference to histological types. *Scand. J. Gastroenterol.*, 13, Suppl. 50, 1978.
19. **Palli, D., Bianchi, S., Decarli, A., Cipriani, F., Avellini, C., Cocco, P., Falcini, F., Puntoni, R., Russo, A., Vindigni, C., Fraumeni, J. F., Jr., Blot, W. J., and Buiatti, E.,** A case-control study of cancers of the gastric cardia in Italy. *Br. J. Cancer*, 65, 263, 1992.
20. **Alberts, S. R., Lanier, A. P., McMahon. B. J., Harpster, A., Bulkow, L., R., Heyward, W. L., and Murray, C.,** Clustering of hepatocellular carcinoma in Alaska native families. *Genet. Epidemiol.*, 8, 127, 1991.
21. **Haddock, G. and Carter, D. C.,** Aetiology of pancreatic cancer. *Br. J. Surg.*, 77, 1159, 1990.
22. **Lynch, H. T., Lanspa, S. J., Fitzgibbons, R.J., Jr., Smyrk, T., Fitzimmons, M. L., and McLellan, J.,** Familial cancer (Part 1): Genetic pathology review. *Neb. Med. J.*, May 1989, page 109.
23. **Lynch, H. T., Fitzimmons, M. L., Smyrk, T. C., et al.** Familial pancreatic cancer: clinicopathologic study of 18 nuclear families. *Am. J. Gastroenterol.*, 85, 54, 1990.
24. **Black, W. C., Key, C. R., Carmany, T. B., and Herman D.,** Carcinoma of the gallbladder in a population of southwestern American Indians. *Cancer*, 39, 1267, 1977.

25. **Devor, E. J. and Buechley R. W.,** Gallbladder cancer in Hispanic New Mexicans. II. Familial occurrence in two northern New Mexico kindreds. *Cancer Genet. Cytogenet.*, 1, 139, 1979.
26. **Trajber, H. J., Szego, T., de Camargo, S.A.H., Jr, H., Mester, M., Marujo, W. C., and Roll, S.,** Adenocarcinoma of the gallbladder in two siblings. *Cancer,* 50, 1200, 1982.
27. **Sperling, M. J.,** Familial biliary tract carcinoma. *J. Am. Med. Assoc.,* 190, 166, 1964.
28. **Lynch, H. T., Ens, J., Lynch, J. F., and Watson, P.,** Tumor variation in three extended Lynch syndrome II kindreds. *Am. J. Gastroenterol.,* 83, 741, 1988.
29. **Mecklin, J.-P., Järvinen, H. J., and Virolainen, M.,** The association between cholangiocarcinoma and hereditary nonpolyposis colorectal carcinoma. *Cancer,* 69, 1112, 1992.
30. **Selby, J. V., Friedman, G. D., Quesenberry, C. P., and Weiss, N. S.,** A case-control study of screening sigmoidoscopy and mortality from colorectal cancer. *N. Engl. J. Med.,* 326, 653, 1992.
31. **Newcomb, P. A., Norfleet, R. G., Storer, B. E., Surawicz, T. S., and Marcus, P. M.,** Screening sigmoidoscopy and colorectal cancer mortality. *J. Natl. Cancer Inst.,* 84, 1572, 1992.
32. **Lynch, H. T., Kimberling, W., Albano, W. A., Lynch, J. F, Biscone, K., Schuelke, G. S., Sandberg, A. A., Lipkin, M., Deschner, E. E., Mikol, Y. B., Elston, R. C., Bailey-Wilson, J. E., and Danes, B. S.,** Hereditary nonpolyposis colorectal cancer. Part I. Clinical description of resource, *Cancer,* 56, 934, 1985.
33. **Mecklin, J.-P.,** Frequency of hereditary colorectal carcinoma. *Gastroenterology,* 93, 1021–1025, 1987.
34. **Lynch, H. T., Smyrk, T., Watson, P., Lanspa, S. J., Boman, B. M., Lynch, P. M., Lynch, J. F., and Cavalieri, J.,** Hereditary colorectal cancer. *Semin. Oncol.,* 18, 337, 1991.
35. **Lynch, H. T. and Lynch J. F.,** The Lynch syndromes. *Curr. Opinion Oncol.,* 5, 687, 1993.
36. **Vasen, H. F., Mecklin, J.-P., Watson, P., Utsunomiya, J., Bertario, L., Lynch, P., Svendsen, L. B., Cristofaro, G., Müller, H., Meera Khan, P., and Lynch, H. T.,** Surveillance in hereditary nonpolyposis colorectal cancer. An international cooperative study of 165 families. *Dis. Colon Rectum,* 36, 1, 1993.
37. **Hakala, T., Mecklin, J.-P., Forss, M., Järvinen, H., and Lehtovirta, P.,** Endometrial carcinoma in the cancer family syndrome. *Cancer,* 68, 1656, 1991.
38. **Peltomäki, P., Aaltonen, L. A., Sistonen P., Pylkänen, L., Mecklin, J.-P., Järvinen, H., Green, J. S., Jass, J. R., Weber, J. L., Leach, F. S., Petersen, G. M., Hamilton, S. R., de la Chapelle, A., and Vogelstein, B.,** Genetic mapping of a locus predisposing to human colorectal cancer. *Science,* 260, 810, 1993.
39. **Lindblom, A., Tannergård, P., Werelius, B., and Nordenskjöld, M.,** Genetic mapping of a second locus predisposing to hereditary non-polyposis colon cancer. *Nat. Genet.,* 5, 279, 1993.
40. **Maher, E. R., Yates, J. R. W., Harries, R., et al.,** Clinical features and natural history of von Hippel-Lindau disease. *Q. J. Med.,* 77, 1151, 1990.
41. **Holman, C. D. J., and Armstrong,** Pigmentary traits, ethnic origin, benign nevi and family as risk factors for cutaneous malignant melanoma. *J. Natl. Cancer Inst.,* 72, 257, 1984.
42. **Clark, W. H., Jr., Elder, D. G., Guerry D., IV, et al.,** A study of tumor progression. The precursor lesions of superficial spreading and nodular melanoma. *Hum. Pathol.,* 15, 732, 1984.
43. **Nobori, T., Miura, K., Wu, D. L., et al.,** Deletions of the cyclin-dependent kinase-4 inhibitor gene in multiple human cancers. *Nature,* 368, 753–755, 1994.
44. **Houlston, R.S ., Murday, V., Harocopos, C., Williams, C. B., and Slack, J.,** Screening and genetic counselling for relatives of patients with colorectal cancer in a family cancer clinic. *BMJ,* 301, 366, 1990.

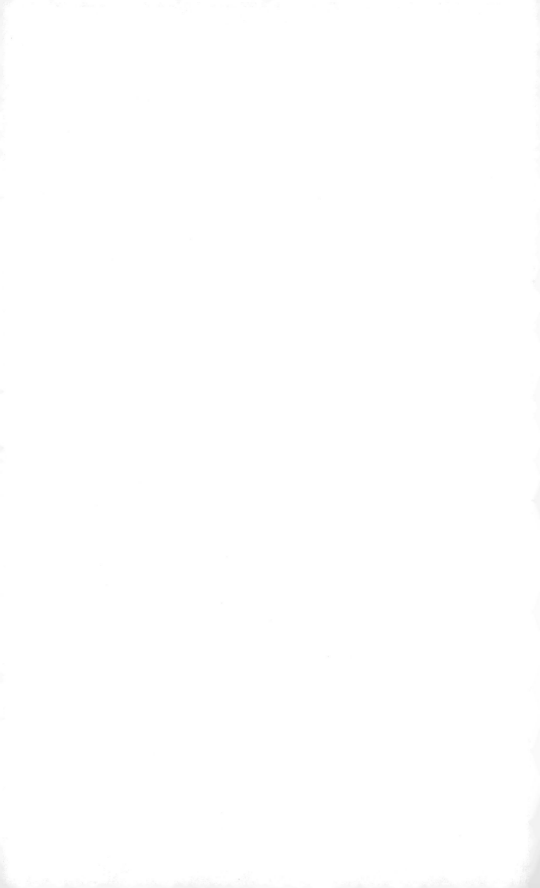

Chapter 11

CHEMOPREVENTION IN FAMILIAL CANCER

Walter Weber

CONTENTS

I. DEFINITION

Chemoprevention of cancer can be defined as the use of noncytotoxic nutrients or pharmacological agents to enhance intrinsic physiological mechanisms that protect the organism against the development and progression of mutant clones of malignant cells.[1] As opposed to chemotherapy of invasive cancer, which kills cancer cells, chemoprevention attempts either to block the initiation of the carcinogenic process or to arrest or reverse the progression of premalignant cells during the long latency period of human cancers. *Chemoprevention of cancer is still an investigational approach.* This chapter does not include food compounds ingested as normal diet; e.g., β-carotene consumed in fruits and vegetables. When extracted and given in specific concentrated pill form, β-carotene falls within the definition of chemoprevention.

II. RATIONALE AND HISTORY

With the aging of the population, cancer mortality is increasing. Cancer treatment is making progress steadily but slowly. Therefore, the therapy for late disease needs to be complemented by other approaches. In recent years, the possibility has been raised that nutritional modification or pharmacological agents can prevent the development of human neoplasia, slow down its progression, or make it regress. Basic research has corroborated this concept.[2]

0-8493-4782-3/96/$0.00+$.50
© 1996 by CRC Press Inc.

Randomized clinical trials over the last 5 years have produced significant activity in reversing oral, skin, colorectal, and cervical premalignancy; in preventing primary skin and stomach cancer; and in preventing second primary tumors associated with head and neck and lung cancer.[3] The initial choice of chemopreventive agents for clinical trials has been limited to a few compounds. It has been dictated by epidemiological and laboratory data available in the late 1970s and by the rigid requirement of the use of a "safe" compound in normal or nearly normal populations.[4]

III. STUDY POPULATIONS

The choice of the study population has important implications. Some researchers choose to study chemoprevention in the setting of primary disease prevention. These *primary prevention trials* are well suited for studying compounds that have the potential health benefits extending beyond a single disease or organ system.[5] The logistical problems in performing these trials are considerable, as they require very large sample sizes and long study durations.[6] Other researchers choose to *study individuals at increased cancer risk*, based on the presence of a premalignant lesion, a history of cancer, or a family history of cancer. This approach concentrates on populations most likely to benefit. But it may be difficult to generalize the findings to a population that does not share the high risk factors. The *safety level* required for chemoprevention should be related to the level of risk.[7] For example, if the study population is composed of normal or nearly normal subjects (such as volunteers with a history of one polyp), very few or no side effects will be tolerated by either subjects or staff. In contrast, if the subjects are at high risk (e.g., have a history of familial polyposis, or second tumors), considerable side effects may be acceptable.

IV. CHEMOPREVENTION BY FAMILY HISTORY — TRIAL RESULTS

Apart from age, a family history of cancer represents one of the most important risk factors for developing cancer, usually of the same localization. The order of magnitude of familial cancer aggregation has about a two- to threefold greater frequency of cancer among relatives of patients than among those of controls.[8-11] To date, *results of randomized trials* are available only for familial colorectal cancer. The agents studied are vitamin C, calcium, and nonsteroidal anti-inflammatory drugs.[3] There are now five randomized trials with low patient numbers that have been completed in familial adenomatous polyposis (Table 1). The designs have used two intermediate endpoints: adenomatous polyp changes and mucosal proliferation changes. The first two studies investigated the activity of vitamin C (ascorbic acid), and vitamin C plus E (α-tocopherol) plus wheat fiber.[12,13] The first study found a reduction in

TABLE 1
Chemoprevention Completed Familial Colorectal Cancer Randomized Trials

First Author (year)	Study Setting	Design (phase)	No. of Patients	Intervention	Outcome[1]
Bussey 1982	FAP[2]	2	36	Vitamin C (3 g/d) vs. placebo	Positive (polyps)
De Cosse 1989	FAP	2	58	Vitamins C(4 g/d), E(400 mg/d) and fiber (22.5 g/d) vs. placebo	Positive (polyps[3])
Stern 1990	Prior FAP	2	31	Calcium (1200 mg/d) vs. placebo	Negative (labeling index)
Labayle 1991	FAP	2	10	Sulindac (300 mg/d) vs. placebo	Positive (polyps)
Giardiello 1993	FAP	2	22	Sulindac (300 mg/d) vs. placebo	Positive (polyps)

[1] Positive = intervention is significantly more active than the control.
[2] FAP = familial adenomatous polyposis.
[3] Significant after adjustment for compliance.

polyp area in the ascorbic acid-treated group (3 g/day) at nine months of follow-up.[12] The second study revealed that the number of polyps decreased under ascorbic acid (4 g/day) plus α-tocopherol (400 mg/day) plus a high wheat fiber supplement (22.5 g/day).[13] The same regimen of vitamins plus a low wheat fiber supplement (2.2 g/day) had no effect.

Calcium supplementation (1.2 g/day) had no effect on cell proliferation in the third trial.[14] Sulindac, a nonsteroidal anti-inflammatory drug (NSAID), 300 mg/day, achieved a decrease in polyp number when given for four months,[15] and in polyp number plus polyp diameter when given for nine months.[16] No patient had complete resolution of polyps. Three months after treatment with sulindac was stopped, both the number and the size of the polyps increased in the sulindac-treated patients but remained lower than the values at baseline. The long-term efficacy and toxicity of sulindac remain to be determined. This drug is unlikely to replace colectomy as standard primary therapy.

Ongoing randomized trials concentrate on familial breast cancer.[3] A trial of 5 years of tamoxifen (20 mg/day) or placebo is currently being coordinated in the U.K. including healthy women aged 45–65 years with one or more of the following:

1. Breast cancer in mother, sister, or daughter diagnosed under the age of 50 years;
2. Mother, sister, or daughter with bilateral breast cancer;
3. Breast cancer in two first- or second-degree relatives;

4. Nulliparous, with a mother or sister with breast cancer;
5. Having had a benign biopsy with proliferative disease, and a mother, sister, or daughter with breast cancer.[17]

Women aged 35–44 will also be eligible if they have

1. A mother or sister diagnosed with cancer in both breasts under the age of 40 years;
2. Two relatives (mother, sisters, or daughters) with breast cancer under the age of 50 years.

This will be an international trial with participation from the U.K., The Netherlands, France, Germany, Switzerland, Australia, New Zealand, and other countries.

The National Surgical Adjuvant Project for Breast and Bowel Cancer (NSABP) in the U.S. has begun a trial designed to enroll 16,000 women (35–78 years old) who are at twofold or greater risk of breast cancer than are women in the general population.[3] The risk, dependent on family history, etc., is assessed by use of the mathematical model reported by Gail et al.[18] This model accurately predicts risk in women with a family history of breast cancer who receive annual mammograms.[19] Tamoxifen's potential beneficial effects on women subjects' cardiovascular and skeletal systems will be evaluated systematically by the NSABP. Strong preclinical *in vivo* data indicate the potential clinical activity of *combined tamoxifen and fenretinide* in preventing breast cancer.[3] Therefore, a multicenter phase III U.S. breast cancer adjuvant chemoprevention trial has recently been designed to evaluate this combination in postmenopausal node-positive women.[3]

Small nonrandomized trials are done in rare hereditary disorders. In one such study, five *xeroderma pigmentosum* patients with extraordinarily increased risk for the development of basal cell skin cancer were studied.[20] In this group, a significant reduction in the number of skin cancers was observed in association with 2 years of high-dose isotretinoin (2 mg/kg/d) treatment. This effect was dose related.[21] The beneficial effect was lost after cessation of the chemopreventive agent.[20] This suggests that isotretinoin is acting at a late stage in the carcinogenic process.

V. OUTLOOK

Chemoprevention is a promising new strategy for reducing the morbidity and mortality of malignancies.[22] Encouraging first results have emerged with ascorbic acid and sulindac in familial adenomatous polyposis and with tamoxifen in familial breast cancer.[3] Chemoprevention must be further evaluated for the ability to prevent cancer at doses with acceptable levels of toxicity. Increasing international collaborations and group formations of familial cancer specialists, each focusing on one familial cancer syndrome, will be ideally suited for running the trials needed.

REFERENCES

1. **Sporn, M. B.,** Chemoprevention of cancer. *Lancet* 342, 1211–1213, 1993.
2. **Bertram, J. S., Kolonel, L., N., and Meyskens, F. L., Jr.,** Rationale and strategies for chemoprevention of cancer in humans. *Cancer Res.* 42: 3012–3031, 1987.
3. **Lippman, S. M., Benner, S. E., and Hong, W. K.,** Cancer chemoprevention. *J. Clin. Oncol.* 12: 851–873, 1994.
4. **Boone, C. W., Kelloff, G. J., and Malone, W. E.,** Identification of candidate cancer chemoprevention agents and their evaluation in animal models and human clinical trials: a review. *Cancer Res.* 50: 2–9, 1990.
5. **Benner, S. E. and Hong, W. K.,** Clinical chemoprevention: developing a cancer prevention strategy. *J. Natl. Cancer Inst.* 85: 1446–1447, 1993.
6. **Zelen, M.,** Are primary cancer prevention trials feasible? *J. Natl. Cancer Inst.* 80: 1442–1444, 1988.
7. **Meyskens, F. L., Jr.,** Coming of age — the chemoprevention of cancer. *N. Engl. J. Med.* 323: 825–827, 1990.
8. **Lilienfeld, A. M.,** Formal discussion of genetic factors in the etiology of cancer: an epidemiologic view. *Cancer Res.* 25, 1330–1335, 1965.
9. **Stephenson, B. M., Murday, V. A., Finan, P. J., and Bishop, D. T.,** Screening for colorectal neoplasia in families. In: *Familial Cancer Control* (Ed. W. Weber) Springer-Verlag, Berlin, 91–94, 1992.
10. **Weber, W.,** Cancer control by family history, *Anticancer Res.* 13: 1197–1202, 1993.
11. **Vogel, V. C., Yeomans, A., and Higginbotham, E.,** Clinical management of women at increased risk for breast cancer. *Breast Cancer Res. Treat.* 28: 195–210, 1993.
12. **Bussey, H. J. R., De Cosse, J. J., Deschner, E. E., et al.** A randomized trial of ascorbic acid in polyposis coli. *Cancer* 50, 1434–1439, 1982.
13. **De Cosse, J. J., Miller, H. H., and Lesser, M. L.,** Effect of wheat fiber and vitamins C and E on rectal polyps in patients with familial adenomatous polyposis. *J. Natl. Cancer Inst.* 81: 1290–1297, 1989.
14. **Stern H. S., Gregoire, R. C., Kashtan, H., et al.** Long-term effects of dietary calcium on risk markers for colon cancer in patients with familial polyposis. *Surgery* 108: 528–533, 1990.
15. **Labayle, D., Fischer, D., Vielh, P., et al.** Sulindac causes regression of rectal polyps in familial adenomatous polyposis. *Gastroenterology* 101: 635–639, 1991.
16. **Giardiello, F. M., Hamilton, S. R., Krush, A. J., et al.** Treatment of colonic and rectal adenomas with sulindac in familial adenomatous polyposis. *N. Engl. J. Med.* 328: 1313–1316, 1993.
17. **Cuzick, J.,** Tamoxifen Prevential Trial. A multicentre trial to evaluate the prevention of breast cancer in high risk women, ICRF Protocol, P.O. Box 123, Lincoln's Inn Fields, London WC2A3PX, pp 1–18, 1992.
18. **Gail, M. H., Brinton, L. A., Byar, D. P., et al.** Projecting individualized probabilities of developing breast cancer for white females who are being examined annually. *J. Natl. Cancer Inst.* 81: 1879–1886, 1989.

19. **Bondy, M. L., Lustbader, E. D., Halabi, S., Ross, E., and Vogel, V. E.,** Validation of a breast cancer risk assessment model in women with a positive family history. *J. Natl. Cancer Inst.* 86: 620–625, 1994.

20. **Kraemer, K. H., Di Giovanna, J. J., Moshell, A. N., et al.** Prevention of skin cancer in xeroderma pigmentosum with the use of oral isotretinoin. *N. Engl. J. Med.* 318: 1633–1637, 1988.

21. **Kraemer, K. H., Di Giovanna, J. J., and Peck, G. L.,** Oral isotretinoin prevention of skin cancer in xeroderma pigmentosum. Individual variation in dose response. *J. Invest. Dermatol.* 94: 544, 1990.

22. **Greenwald, P., Kellogg, G., Busch-Whitman, C., and Kramer, B. S.,** Chemoprevention. *CA* 45: 31–49, 1995.

Chapter 12

THE ROLE OF THE NURSE IN FAMILIAL CANCER

Hans-Rudolf Stoll

CONTENTS

I. INTRODUCTION

That certain cancers occur unexpectedly (meaning more than normally in the population) in specific families has been known for many years (e.g., stomach cancer in Napoleon's family; Weber et al., 1990). To meet the special needs of such families, interdisciplinary teams have been established by medical doctors for many years in various places. The main directions of research in these families can be summarized into four areas:

1. Identifying the risk(s) (genetic, environmental, chance)
2. Establishing the cause of the elevated risk
3. Offer actions for primary prevention or cure through early detection
4. Counsel people with an increased familial risk (e.g., concerning their reproductive behavior or responsibility in avoiding risks or detecting cancers early)

Nurses have taken on tasks in the field of familial cancer probably from the beginning in the early 1960s. In particular, they work in three different areas:

1. As nurses in running clinics for identifying persons at risk (early detection of breast cancer, cervical cancer, malignant melanoma, and others)
2. As research nurses in supporting medical doctors in their research
3. As nurse researchers in investigating what nursing can contribute for such families

This chapter sets out to identify the potential role of the nurse in all three dimensions mentioned above. Each section will be supported by a deliberate selection of literature. This is done — due to the title of this chapter — mainly by mentioning nurses. It is, however, as will be shown at the end of this chapter, impossible to run a familial cancer clinic without very close cooperation of a whole range of professions.

II. NURSING CARE

Two main areas seem to emerge from the literature where nurses play an active role in the direct care of clients with an increased risk for cancer:

- Communicating (teaching and counselling) with the clients
- Collecting and managing data (pedigree, blood and tissue samples)

It is often the nurse who establishes the first contact with the client and she is also often the first to see them at the place and time of choice (e.g., the evening at the client's home) (Skirton, 1994). Nurses are in a special position to draw together the meaning of the risk for a specific cancer and the consequences this has, and can discuss these in the background of the familial circumstances with the client in his/her particular situation (Frets, 1990; Skirton, 1994). Nurses also often seem to be involved in teaching the client concerning early signs of cancer or suggested changes in behavior (Fraser, 1982). Müller (1985) states that there is a tremendous need for counselling the clients since there are very few people who have knowledge and skill in this task. Counselling consists of telling the accurate diagnosis, determining risks, and commnnicating the genetic and medical facts, combined with the evaluation of the options and alternatives available (Müller 1990,1992). However, counselling clearly involves more than facts. It includes helping the individuals involved to understand the meaning of the facts and helping them learn to cope with this diagnosis and its implications (Skirton, 1994, Stoll, 1992, Buddeberg, 1981).

Concerning the management of data, it is often the nurse's task to assemble the families, take all data in order to draw the pedigree, take blood and tissue samples, and keep the records of the collected samples (Houlston, 1990; Mulvihill, 1993). However, it is important to know that the actual tasks or the selection thereof carried out by a nurse varies with each nurse working in a particular clinic. There is a lack of nationally accepted job descriptions for such nurses (Skirton, 1994).

III. RESEARCH NURSE

Nurses have always been actively involved in the clinical research of their medical colleagues. This role of supporting others in their research is called a research nurse. They usually work on two distinctive levels:

- Data collection and data management
- Administration of the therapy or control of patients on trial

Increasingly, medical teams have a nurse whose major task is to ensure that doctors fill in the necessary forms correctly and in time. They coordinate and manage the data. But nurses are also involved in the administration of drugs and the monitering of patients for side effects. This important task is increasingly recognised in that nurses are often included as coauthors in medical publications. In familial cancer it is often the nurses who check individuals for early signs of cancer (Fraser, 1982).

IV. NURSING RESEARCH

The role of the nurses in assisting medical doctors in their research is possibly as old as the nursing profession. However, despite the fact that nurses such as Florence Nightingale have carried out their own research, nursing research has only more recently been recognized as a field of its own. The overall goal of nursing research is to increase the knowledge in nursing by systematic enquiry. Little is known, e.g., about the effect that counselling has in these individuals, what information is meaningful to these clients, and what is probably important for the counselling team. By which means could compliance be improved? How could a family cancer clinic be run effectively? In its paper about interdisciplinary collaborative studies in the genetic epidemiology of cancer (National Cancer Institute, 1993), one component that should be studied is "Studies to evaluate the potential benefits, risks and psychological impact of testing and counselling for individuals at increased risk to develop cancer and their families." It would be paramount for nurses to direct efforts in this field. A similar list has been compiled by the U.S. Institutes of Health about research in familial cancer.

REFERENCES

Buddeberg, C., 1981, Krebserkrankung und Familie, *Schweiz. Rundsch. Med. (Praxis)*, 70, 985, 987.

Fraser, M. C., 1982, The role of the nurse in the prevention and early detection of malignant melanoma, *Cancer Nursing*, 5, 351–360.

Frets, P. G., 1990, Factors influencing the reproductive decision after genetic counselling, *Am. J. Med. Genet.*, 35, 496–562.

Houlston, R. S., Murday, V., Haracopos, C., Williams, C. B., and Slack, J., 1990, Screening and genetic counselling for relatives of patients with colorectal cancer in a family cancer clinic, *Br. Med. J.*, 301, 366–368.

Müller, H., 1985, Familial cancer in Basel: some aspects, In Müller, H. and Weber, W. (Eds.) *Familial Cancer*, S. Karger, London.

Müller H., 1990, Genetic counselling and cancer, In Weber, W., Laffer, U., and Durig, M., (Eds.): *Heriditary Cancer and Preventive Surgery*, S. Karger, Basel.

Müller, H., 1992, Cancer Prevention through genetic counselling, in Weber, W. (Ed.), *Familial Cancer Control*, Springer-Verlag, New York.

Mulvihill, J. J., 1993, Genetic counselling of the cancer patient, In DeVita, V., Jr., Hellmann, S., and Rosenberg, S. A., (Ed.): *Cancer Principles and Practice of Oncology*, 4th ed. J.B. Lippincott, Philadelphia.

National Cancer Institute, 1993, Interdisciplinary collaborative studies in the genetic epidemiology of cancer, NIH Guide, 22, 15, April 16.

Skirton, H., 1994, More than an information service? — Should genetic service offer client counselling?, *Prof. Nurse*, 9, 6, (March) 400–404.

Stoll, H., 1992, The nurse's role in familial cancer, in Weber, W. (Ed.), *Familial Cancer Control*, Springer-Verlag, New York.

Tucker, M. A., Fraser, M. C., Goldstein, A. M., Elder, D. A., DuPont, G. IV., and Organic, S. M., 1993, Risk of melanoma and other cancers in melanoma-prone families, *J. Invest. Dermatol.*, 100, 3, Suppl. 350S–355S.

Weber, W., Laffer, U., and Durig, M., (Eds.), 1990, *Hereditary Cancer and Preventive Surgery*, S. Karger. Basel.

Chapter 13

ETHICAL ISSUES

Raanan Gillon

CONTENTS

0-8493-4782-3/96/$0.00+$.50
© 1996 by CRC Press Inc.

I. INTRODUCTION

All the standard problems of ordinary medical practice arise in the context of management of familial cancer. In addition, it is an area of medicine that paradigmatically straddles the interface between ordinary therapeutic medical practice concerned with individual patients on the one hand, and types of medical practice that are orientated to groups and populations on the other — notably medical research, epidemiology, and public health. Thus, management of family cancer is confronted by a series of ethical synergies where the interests of the individual and of the group coincide, but also by ethical tensions when the interests of the individual patient conflict with the interests of others, whether these are other members of the patient's family, potential future beneficiaries of medical research, or the public at large seeking better control of the scourge of cancer.

Among the multifold problems of medical ethics that may potentially arise in the context of medical management of familial cancer, some are particularly relevant. They include issues of adequately informed consent; confidentiality where other members of a potentially affected family may be affected by such confidentiality; benignly intended medical deception and withholding of information, for example, when unsought and potentially distressing or damaging information is discovered; nondirective vs. directive or persuasive counseling; problems in risk benefit assessment including problems associated with probability, and problems that arise when the beneficiaries and the risk takers are different people; problems of inadequate resources for familial cancer management; problems of conflicting rights; legal aspects (dealt with in Chapter 14); ethical issues associated specifically with screening and especially with genetic screening, including implications for the individual in relation to medical insurance, to employment, and to the problem of social stigmatization that a label of 'genetic inferiority' may cause; the ethical problems of prenatal diagnosis; the ethical problems associated with genetic manipulation, including the potential problems of genetic therapy, both somatic and germ-line.

II. A MEDICO-MORAL ANALYTIC FRAMEWORK

In reviewing the ethical issues associated with family cancer management, I shall use an analytic framework developed by Beauchamp and Childress[1] and outlined more briefly in my own book,[2] based on four *prima facie* moral obligations which almost everyone accepts regardless of religion, politics, culture, or philosophical presuppositions, along with attention to the scope of application of these principles (to whom or to what do we owe these obligations?). The principles are

- **Respect for people's autonomy** — for their deliberated decisions for themselves — in so far as such respect is compatible with equal respect for the autonomy of all those potentially affected.

- **Beneficence** — an obligation to benefit others.
- **Non-maleficence** — an obligation not to harm others.
- **Justice** — an obligation to be fair, whether in the contexts of distribution of scarce resources, respect for people's rights, or respect for morally acceptable laws.

Prima facie, a term introduced by the Oxford philosopher David Ross, means that the principle is morally binding unless it conflicts with another moral principle, in which case one has to choose between the competing moral principles. The four-principles-plus scope approach does not provide a decision method for choosing between conflicting principles. It does however provide a basic common moral commitment, a basic common moral language, and a basic cross-cultural approach to thinking more clearly about our moral obligations.

III. RESPECT FOR AUTONOMY IN THE MANAGEMENT OF FAMILIAL CANCER

A. ADEQUATELY INFORMED CONSENT

As with all medical interventions on autonomous agents, the adequately informed consent of the patient is a prerequisite if the patient's autonomy is to be respected, no matter what the proposed intervention is to be. Just as in standard cancer care, whether curative or palliative, adequately informed consent is these days considered the moral norm,[3-5] so, whether the proposal is for genetic screening, genetic testing, prenatal testing, or even genetic counseling itself, if we are to respect the patient's autonomy sufficient information must be given for the patient to be able to make an autonomous decision about whether or not to accept the offer of intervention.

B. MEDICAL CONFIDENTIALITY

One of the most venerable of medico-moral obligations, explicitly required of doctors in the Hippocratic Oath, medical confidentiality can be justified on the moral grounds both of respecting patients' autonomy and of welfare maximization.[2]

Nonetheless, though it is a very strong moral obligation, medical confidentiality is not generally regarded, *pace* Kottow,[6] as an absolute moral obligation, and indeed probably was not regarded as absolute in the Hippocratic Oath itself. Sufficiently important competing moral concerns may, it is widely accepted, justify the breaking of medical confidences. For example, in the U.K. the General Medical Council (GMC), which has overriding control over professional medical ethics, and is able to withdraw doctors' licenses to practice medicine if they are guilty of seriously unethical conduct, accepts several exceptions to the rule of confidentiality.[7] These include statutory obligations such as those relating to notification of infectious disease, abortion, and the prevention of terrorism; obligations to obey the instructions of a judge to divulge confidential information; inspection of records for the purposes of bona fide medical research approved by a research ethics committee; and, rarely, when the public interest overrides the duty of confidentiality as, for example, when requested to assist the police in the investigation of a grave or serious crime. And in the case of HIV infection the GMC recognizes that it may be ethically justifiable to override the obligation of confidentiality to one patient in order to try to protect the life of another.[7]

Knowledge that a person's disease has a genetic basis is obviously of potential relevance to the lives and health of other members of the person's family, but sometimes patients or clients refuse to allow such genetic information to be passed on to family members. In the U.S., the President's Commission on Bioethics recommended that confidentiality could be justifiably over-ridden in the context of genetic disorders if several conditions were met.[8] First, efforts had to be made to encourage the patient or client to disclose the genetic information himself or herself, or to give permission to the doctor to disclose it. Second, there had to be a high probability both that without such disclosure harm would occur and that the information disclosed would be used to avert the harm. Third, the harm would be serious and would be suffered by identifiable individuals. Fourth, precautions would be taken to ensure that only genetic information needed for diagnosis and/or treatment of the disease in question would be disclosed.

Ten years later, in the U.K., the Nuffield Council on Bioethics also recommended that in exceptional circumstances it would be justifiable for doctors to override confidentiality where efforts to persuade the patient to disclose relevant genetic information had been rejected and where non-disclosure would be "potentially damaging rather than merely inconvenient" for other family members. The Nuffield Council also recommended that a patient's malicious refusal to permit disclosure of genetic information to family members might also justify overriding confidentiality. The Council reiterated the general importance of medical confidentiality and urged professional organizations to prepare guidelines concerning those exceptional cases where overriding confidentiality might be justified.[9]

C. BENIGNLY INTENDED DECEPTION AND WITHHOLDING OF INFORMATION

Just as in other areas of medical practice, moral dilemmas may arise in the management of familial cancer concerning whether or not to deceive a patient or to withhold information. As with maintenance of confidentiality, there are in general strong *prima facie* medico-moral obligations not to deceive patients and not to withhold information from them — possession of which they would wish to have.[2]

However, cases will arise in which deceit and or nondisclosure are morally justified, notably those in which the patient or client would want the doctor's deceit or nondisclosure. Take two examples: at least some patients would not wish to discover that they had testicular feminization syndrome (androgen insensitivity syndrome), i.e., they would not want to be told that they were chromosomally male despite having entirely female secondary sexual characteristics. They are likely to have been brought up as females, they may have married, and they have usually come to the doctor for investigation of infertility. The diagnosis explains their infertility. In addition, their residual undescended testicular tissue poses a risk of cancer if it is not excised.[10] Yet while some patients would wish to be told the full details, however distressing, others would prefer to be deceived and/or have information withheld.

Or take the example of unanticipated additional findings such as nonpaternity (an incidental finding in about 2% of one series in Oxford[11]). Some would wish to be told — others would not — that they are not the genetic offspring of their parent (usually father), or that they are not the genetic father of their child.

As with so many moral dilemmas in medicine, there are no straightforwardly right answers in such cases. However, the problems can presumably be diminished (a) by asking people in advance how they would wish to be treated in the event of various hypothetical eventualities, and (b) by indicating in advance how the doctor or clinic concerned would normally respond in the event of various eventualities, unless requested to respond differently. In such ways, the views of the individuals concerned are more likely to approximate, with resulting mutual agreement about the best way to act. (In addition, prospective empirical studies designed to discover ways of achieving mutually ethically acceptable outcomes would seem to be desirable.)

D. TO PERSUADE, OR EVEN TO INSIST?

One of the widely agreed norms of genetic counseling is that it should be nondirective.[12] Respect for the patient's autonomy requires that the doctor who wishes to benefit the patient provides information and advice, but that it is for the patient or client to decide what to do, after taking into account that information and advice. While this undoubtedly remains the norm, as indicated above, some argue that there are cases where attempts may be morally justifiable to persuade patients to act in one way rather than another, and even — in rare cases where serious harm to others can be averted — to override the patient's own decision to withhold genetic information from potentially affected family members. In such cases, the benefit of preventing harm to others by passing on potentially lifesaving genetic information is regarded as morally even more important than respecting the patient's or client's autonomous decision that the information should be withheld.

For example, if genetic screening shows that other family members may be at risk of inherited colon cancer or inherited breast cancer, many would feel that those family members should be informed and thus given the opportunity to take potentially lifesaving action to reduce their risk. Some would feel that the family members should be informed even if the index patient refused permission to divulge the relevant genetic information.

Once again there seems to be no clear cut Right Answer in such dilemmas, answers to which depend either on the relative weight or importance given to the conflicting moral principles or on differing assessments of the amount of harm and benefit that would result from different moral policies. Thus some would give greater weight to respect for autonomy, and insist on preserving absolute or near absolute confidentiality, perhaps also arguing that overall welfare would be maximized by doing so. Others would reason that preventing serious harm to family members was morally more important than respecting the patient's autonomy by maintaining confidentiality. And where such genetic screening programs were being paid for by others than the client, for example by national health systems or by charitable organizations, or by mutual health insurance systems, the funders might add that justice in meeting the serious medical needs of others was morally more important than maintaining the patient's confidentiality at the cost of serious potential and preventable harm to those others.

One approach that would seem at least to reduce the moral problems of such dilemmas would, once again, be to make clear in advance what the approach of the doctor or clinic concerned would actually be. Would absolute or near absolute confidentiality be maintained or would information be transmitted to family members in cases where such transmission would avert serious harm to those family members, even against the patient's instructions to the contrary? And if the latter, then perhaps agreement to such disclosure should be made a condition of participation in genetic testing, as the U.S. President's Commission on Bioethics suggested.[8] At least that way patients or clients seeking or being offered genetic testing would understand the implications of participation, and would be in a position to decline to participate if they found such implications unacceptable.

IV. BENEFITS AND HARMS IN THE MANAGEMENT OF FAMILIAL CANCER

The fundamental moral objective of doctors has been, at least since Hippocratic times, to produce net medical benefit-over-harm for their patients. However this formulation is ambiguous between benefit for the particular patient — the patient being cared for at the moment — and benefit for patients more generally. Typically, for the ordinary 'treating doctor' — for example, the hospital doctor taking in emergency patients or the general medical practitioner seeing patients in the surgery — the needs of the individual patient take moral precedence over the needs of groups of patients. However, once the doctor becomes involved with medical research or with epidemiology or with population medicine, the balance changes, and the needs of the individual patient become subsumed in the needs of others — future patients or other groups or populations. Both types of activity are undoubtedly beneficial, but it is important to be clear which activity is being pursued at any time and to make this clear to the patient. This is particularly important if any risk or even inconvenience is being proposed for the patient that is not for that patient's benefit but for the potential benefit of others.

It is particularly important because the basic assumption of the therapeutic doctor-patient relationship — the "social contract" between patients and their doctors — is that unless otherwise specified any risk of harm or even of nuisance or inconvenience proposed by the doctor will only be proposed if, in the doctor's professional opinion, it is in the patient's interests to undergo that risk. Every knife cut is a harm, but a patient can trust a doctor to propose surgery only if, in the doctor's professional opinion, surgery will produce a net medical benefit for that patient, with minimal harm. If the doctor proposed the surgery because he was doing a research project of no medical relevance to the patient, then of course he would have to explain that the normal therapeutic relationship was irrelevant to the proposal and he was merely asking the patient to participate in a nontherapeutic research project which, it was hoped, would be of medical benefit to others in the future.

Family cancer management typically involves medical interventions aimed *both* at benefiting the individual patient *and* at benefiting other members of the patient's family. In addition, insofar as it often also includes extensive research involvement, both into the epidemiology and into the medical management of the relevant cancers, there is also an objective of benefiting not only the patient and his or her family but also other patients and potential patients in the future. For any proposed intervention it is morally important to distinguish, so far as is possible, between these various objectives and to make them as clear as possible to the patient.

For example, mammography for a woman who has a strong family history of breast cancer is generally offered entirely in the interests of that individual woman. The harms and benefits of early detection in general and mammography in particular are explained just as for any other early diagnostic intervention, including the notion of her increased risk of cancer because of the potential genetic linkage. The mammography is done only if the woman accepts that, overall, it would be beneficial for her.

Suppose intraductal carcinoma *in situ* is discovered as a result of that mammography, and the patient's doctor wishes (a) to recruit her into a prospective trial of three different approaches to management of the condition,[13,14] (b) to add her name and details to a cancer registry, and (c) to contact other female relatives for investigation of their breast cancer status. Here the doctor is adding to the traditional therapeutic concern for the individual patient a concern for the medical welfare of others. Few would doubt that such concern is anything other than admirable, but it is a different and broader concern than the traditional Hippocratic concern to benefit the individual patient, and insofar as it involves the patient in any risk of harm, nuisance, or inconvenience that is not directly in her interests, this ought to be made clear to her and her consent obtained, and her refusal to consent respected.

Most patients are happy to consent to such proposals when they are based on good reasons which are clearly and helpfully explained. However, some may not wish to participate for their own reasons.

A. DISAGREEMENT BETWEEN PATIENT AND DOCTOR ABOUT HARMS AND BENEFITS

If, despite ample discussion, counseling, and attempts at persuasion in the interests of others, the patient continues to reject any or all of the interventions proposed, there can be little doubt that if her wishes in these contexts were simply overridden she would be harmed, her autonomy would be overridden, her trust in doctors would be undermined, and the current norms of medical ethics would be transgressed. On the other hand, others may well be protected from harm.

Some might argue, as indicated above in the context of making it a condition of genetic investigation and counseling, that relevant information would have to be shared with family members, that the harms to the individual patient of transgressing confidentiality are outweighed by the overall benefits obtained. More good than harm, overall, would be produced, they might argue, if in such cases the patient's views were simply overridden (or she were simply not consulted) and she were recruited into the trial, her name entered on the cancer registry, and relevant family members approached.

A problem with such moral arguments is that they may fail to consider the broader harms that might be anticipated to result from such a policy. For once it became generally known that, without consultation or consent, patients might be recruited into research trials, their details added to computerized registers for follow-up, and medical information about them passed on to members of their families without their consent, trust in doctors and in the institutions of medicine could be expected to plummet. Such trust grounds good medical practice, and without it standards of medical care could be expected to fall drastically, and its costs to soar, as distrustful patients required full information about every proposed intervention before deciding whether or not it was in their interests. As for agreeing to do anything that was not in their direct interests, altruism shrivels under compulsion and agreement to do things to help others could be expected to be generally forthcoming only if it were made legally obligatory. Thus it is not at all clear that overall welfare would be maximized by such a policy, even if overall welfare were agreed to be the sole moral determinant.

B. THE CASE OF PROPHYLACTIC MASTECTOMY

Intermittently, disagreement arises between patients and their doctors about the assessment of potential harms and benefits. The doctor may recommend surgery and chemotherapy as most likely to produce the maximal medical benefit with the least harm, while the patient may find radiotherapy optimal. The doctor may recommend a blood transfusion when for the patient, a Jehovah's

Witness, blood transfusion may constitute a vastly greater harm even than death. In general, the assessment of harms and benefits is in the last resort an intensely personal affair, depending on the individual's own values and approaches to the management of risk — what Fried called a person's "risk budget".[15] Thus the doctor can advise on the objective descriptions of various alternative options, on their probabilities, on how the doctor's experience and or scientific trials have shown that people tend to respond when these various alternatives actually occur, and on what the doctor would advise the patient to choose in the circumstances. Still, the assessment of how harmful and how beneficial the various alternative options are likely to be for a particular patient will depend in large measure on that individual's own evaluation.

An interesting limiting case of potential disagreement between doctor and patient about the harms and benefits of alternative courses of action arises in the case of prophylactic mastectomy for women with a strong family history of breast cancer.[16,17] A small minority of such women may prefer bilateral prophylactic mastectomy to regular breast screening and the continuing risk, and associated anxiety, that despite such screening they will die from a rapidly metastasizing breast cancer that has been detected too late. (The risk of a woman developing breast cancer in the rare familial cases where her mother and one sister have had breast cancer in both breasts is as high as 25% and even higher, 85%, in carriers of *BRCA1* gene mutation.)[17]

A common medical response to the idea of prophylactic mastectomy is amazed disgust that any woman could contemplate such mutilation when it was not necessary. However, this is surely a further example of variation in people's personal assessments of what counts as harms and benefits for themselves, and of their relative importance. Given sufficient personal concern about the increased genetic risk of breast cancer, given sufficient personal value ascribed to its prevention, and given sufficient personal readiness to sacrifice what to many women are such crucial elements of their sense of feminine identity, it is difficult to understand why a doctor should reject a woman's decision to request prophylactic mastectomy. However, it remains the case that many doctors would consider such an operation too mutilatingly harmful, with too small a potential justifying benefit, for them to consider carrying it out themselves. As with cases of abortion, however, while the doctor's autonomy can be respected so too can the patient's — by offering her the opportunity to find a surgeon who would be prepared to carry out her wishes. It would be hard to argue that such a course of action would be so unacceptable to the medical profession or to the public, or so clearly against the public interest, that it required a professional or a legal ban. (By contrast, amputation of a healthy limb at the request of a patient who is keen to avoid military conscription might well be argued to require such a ban, even though the operation might well be in the individual patient's interests!)

V. JUSTICE AND MANAGEMENT OF FAMILIAL CANCER

Ethical considerations of justice apply as much (but no more) to the management of familial cancer as they do to any other aspect of medical practice. In the context of distributive justice — fair distribution of scarce resources — the same sorts of potentially conflicting moral considerations arise as for other aspects of medical practice.[18] Alas no general prescription can be given for what constitutes fair distribution of scarce resources, but some recurring moral themes are worth reiterating. These include the fact that distributive justice involves *competing* moral claims and that not all of these claims can be met. The claims include those of the people with existing and meetable medical needs of different degrees; the claims of those with currently largely unmeetable medical needs (a main concern both of palliative care and of medical research); the claims of those providing the resources (who, among other concerns, will inevitably be keen to avoid waste of those resources, to achieve as much benefit as possible from those resources, and to limit the amount of resources they are required to provide); the claims of those providing the health care (who, among other concerns, will wish to maintain an adequately professional standard of health care and a differential moral concern in favor of their actual patients over the interests of patients in general). Acknowledgment of the moral relevance of all the competing claims relevant to distributive justice, and of their complexity, helps to prevent simplistic acceptance of simplistic solutions. But the stark dilemma of distributive justice in the context of scarce resources is always and inevitably present — none of the legitimate claims may be legitimately ignored, yet by definition not all the legitimate claims can be met.

Issues of justice in relation to rights can be similarly complex. Points worth reiterating in the context of familial cancer management are that widely acknowledged rights of patients, including cancer patients and potential cancer patients, include not only a right to fair distribution of available resources but also, as indicated above, a right not to have their bodies or minds interfered with without their adequately informed consent; a right not to be deceived; a right to have their confidences respected; as well as a right to have treatments that have been professionally assessed to be for them the best available and to produce the most benefit for them with the least possible harm. Of course, as with other aspects of justice, these rights may conflict, but they may be overridden only where a competing moral concern can justifiably be claimed to take precedence.

One important issue of rights in the context of familial cancer, as with all serious genetic disorders, is the question of the rights of fetuses in relation to abortion (for if genetic screening methods were developed to identify genetic cancer predispositions of fetuses *in utero*, as other genetic abnormalities such as Down's syndrome can now be identified, the issue arises of whether abortion of affected fetuses should be morally and legally available to pregnant women). This issue, essentially one of whether fetuses fall within the full scope of our moral obligations to each other, will be considered further below, in the context of stigmatization.

Finally in the context of justice and familial cancer management, legal justice is of considerable importance and is considered in Chapter 14.

VI. ETHICAL PROBLEMS OF GENETIC SCREENING

One of the routine activities in the management of familial cancer is genetic screening. Many of the ethical issues discussed above are relevant to genetic screening, but as such screening is likely to become more widespread, certain ethical issues deserve additional notice. Three of these relate to genetic screening in the context of life and health insurance, in the context of employment, and, more generally, in the context of the social stigmatization of 'genetic inferiority'.

A. INSURANCE
Should insurance companies be allowed to require genetic screening prior to issuing life or health policies? On the one hand such insurance can be regarded as a commercial transaction based on a gamble about disease, disability, or premature death, with the parties free to seek to minimize their risks. Genetic screening from this perspective is simply a potentially more efficient means of risk reduction for the insurer than the currently permitted medical history, which includes information elicited about a client's family medical history precisely in order to reduce the insurer's risk of paying out for inherited disease, disability, or premature death.

On the other hand, medical insurance may be seen as a social obligation that should be provided for all, regardless of their individual risk of disease, disability, and premature death, whether this risk is genetic, environmental, or some combination of the two.

Decisions about whether or not to permit insurance companies to require genetic screening of potential clients will depend on the balance within different societies of these two motivations for medical insurance. Ethically, it seems that both elements are justifiable. However, the more a society's provision of health care to its members, especially its poorer members, is based on medical insurance, the more wary it needs to be if it wishes to fulfill a moral obligation to provide beneficent health care for its members regardless of their risk and regardless of their ability to pay for it. But even in such societies there is no reason to make its medical insurance companies bear *unlimited* risks in relation to genetic disorders. For example, and most obviously, if the potential client is able to obtain genetic screening and knows of a specific genetic defect it is difficult to justify any rule that prevents the medical insurance company having access to the same information.

A "compromise" approach advocated in the U.K.[9] has been to recommend that insurance companies should not require any genetic tests as a prerequisite of insurance; but that for sums above a certain level they should be permitted to require disclosure of any genetic tests already performed. In addition, since it is currently insurance company practice to charge similarly weighted premiums for both a positive family history for a condition and for a positive genetic test for the same condition, it has been recommended that in cases of positive family history of genetic disorders insurance companies should be allowed to require disclosure of any genetic tests already performed, provided they continue not to increase the disadvantage to the client if the test has been positive and provided they treat the client as if he or she had had no family history of the disorder if the test has been negative.

B. EMPLOYMENT

It is already widely accepted that employers may medically screen both potential and actual employees to determine their medical fitness for their proposed or actual employment. The advent of genetic screening and testing makes this potentially highly disadvantageous to individuals if a positive genetic test for a disorder, whether an inherited cancer or Huntington's disease or any other disease that is likely to interfere with working capacity, can be used to justify permanent exclusion from employment or categories of employment. Various competing concerns may encourage such genetic testing. The most obvious is concern of the employer to avoid expense, whether in training costs or in pension costs for early retirement on medical grounds. A second concern is to avoid risk to others. A third concern is to avoid risk to the employee.

Many countries have already banned employment discrimination on the grounds of pregnancy or potential pregnancy, even though such discrimination is undoubtedly of financial benefit to employers. Support for pregnant women is seen in such countries as socially desirable, as is distribution of the burden of such support among employers. Similar reasoning is available in relation to costs of caring for those with a genetic predisposition to health problems. Clearly, the more that employers are able to avoid such costs themselves the more the burden is shifted onto others — either onto the individuals themselves and those who care for them, or onto the state.

As for exclusion from employment on grounds of protecting the health of the employee, both on grounds of respect for the autonomy of the individual and on grounds of individual harm and benefit assessment, it is surely better to allow the employee himself or herself to decide what is most beneficial. A genetic predisposition to some disorder may well be encouraged to express itself by certain sorts of work, but many individuals may find it more beneficial to have the job and the accompanying increased risk than to be excluded from both. Meanwhile, employers should be required to minimize the hazards by reasonable environmental standards.[19]

A substantial risk to others remains a clearly justifiable basis for excluding employees on health grounds; far less clear, however, are examples of genetic predispositions to ill health creating such substantial risks to others; certainly, genetic predispositions to hereditary cancer seem unlikely to do so.

C. SOCIAL STIGMA

The idea that one has a genetic defect is for some people highly distressing and shame-inducing and, correspondingly, the idea that someone else has such a defect can create social stigmatization. While a leg broken in a skiing accident seems widely socially acceptable, perhaps for some even admirable, a leg genetically withered from birth often creates social stigma, rejection, even hostility. Evidence of social stigmatization resulting from genetic screening for sickle cell trait is given in a U.S. Office of Technology Assessment report, which also states that, as a result, laws banning such discrimination and laws banning mandatory sickle cell testing were introduced.[20] On the other hand, it seems possible to introduce genetic screening without social stigmatization.[21] The U.K. Nuffield Council on Bioethics recommends that the dangers of such stigmatization can be reduced by proper educational programs, both for those being genetically tested and for the public at large, from schooldays onwards. And they suggest that part of such education should be to point out that each of us carries a genetic mutation for at least one serious recessive disorder, i.e., we are all "carriers". "If everyone realizes that he or she is a carrier, there can be no stigma."[21]

D. ABORTION FOR GENETIC DEFECT

A major perceived problem of social stigmatization is that of termination of pregnancy for genetic abnormality. Some argue that quite apart from any fundamental moral objection to abortion per se, such termination stigmatizes and devalues people with the relevant abnormalities and, indeed, with genetic abnormalities in general. Such views, widespread and sincere though they may be, are, I believe, based on a logical fallacy — on flawed reasoning.[22] Abortion for fetal abnormality can only be morally acceptable, except where it is done to save the life of the pregnant woman, if the fetus does not have the same moral status as a person. If, as is widely accepted, and morally defensible by any, all, or some combination of the four principles, killing people who are nonaggressors is morally wrong unless in self defense, or at their sustained autonomous request in contexts of irremediable suffering, then to kill a person who is handicapped or disabled is as morally unacceptable as to kill a person who is not so handicapped or disabled. But for those who accept abortion, to kill a fetus, whether it is normal or abnormal, is not to kill a person, for they believe that a fetus does not have the moral status of a person, even though it has the *potential* for developing that status. Thus, for those who accept abortion, fetuses do not fall within the scope of our strong obligation not to kill people. For them, killing a fetus is not killing a person, and may be justifiable, even in the absence of aggression, self defense, or autonomous request, given sufficient benefit. One such sufficient benefit that justifies abortion for many such people (and in many legislations) is to prevent the coming into being of a *person* with a major handicap or disability.

Given acceptance of the fundamental distinction between moral obligations owed to persons and moral obligations owed to entities who are not persons, and given that fetuses are not (yet) persons, there are no logical implications for attitudes to handicapped or disabled persons that stem from acceptance of abortion of fetuses with major abnormalities — just as there are no implications for attitudes to persons without handicap or disability that follow from acceptance of abortion of fetuses that do not have abnormalities. Given the assumptions that justify abortion, it is no more stigmatizing to persons who have handicaps and disabilities to abort fetuses with such handicaps and disabilities than it is stigmatizing to people without handicaps or disabilities to abort fetuses without handicaps and disabilities.

Of course, if the assumption that the fetus has a lesser moral status than a person is rejected, and instead it is assumed that fetuses have or should be given the same moral respect as people, then it clearly follows that fetuses should not be killed on account of handicap or disability, no more than older handicapped and disabled people should be killed on this account. Given the assumption that fetuses are people, or have or should be accorded the same moral status as people, it certainly and obviously would be morally unacceptable discrimination against handicapped and disabled people to allow selective abortion of handicapped and disabled fetuses.

VII. GENETIC MANIPULATION

Many of the moral issues arising in the context of genetic manipulation have already been alluded to above. Several recurring concerns may additionally be worth brief mention, notably concerns that genetic manipulation is "playing god", is "unnatural", (especially trans-species genetic manipulation), and is too dangerous, especially if the genetically manipulated changes can be transmitted to offspring (germ-line therapy).

A. "PLAYING GOD"

Although this is a common criticism, it is difficult to be sure what precisely it amounts to. If the criticism resides in the notion of "playing" then of course interventions that may adversely affect the lives of others are potentially of serious import, and should not be performed "playfully" or as if they are a game. Such an admonition is as important for work in genetic manipulation as it is for any other sort of activity that may adversely affect the lives of others — but there seems no special reason to single out molecular scientists for such admonitions.

If the emphasis is on intervening in a way that was previously impossible for mere humans — so that in that sense the intervention appears arrogantly or "hubristically god-like" — the criticism would prevent *all* new interventions of which humans were previously incapable. All scientific and technological developments, including all the developments of medical science, have appeared "god-like" in this sense, and yet in retrospect have created enormous benefits for mankind, though also of course significant harms. Again, there is an important warning here if what it boils down to is an admonition to be careful and responsible about the potential harms that beneficially intended new developments may cause. But again there seems no special reason to single out genetic manipulation for such a warning — it applies to all new interventions, not just in medical science but in all spheres of human activity intended to benefit others but which may also harm them.

B. "UNNATURAL"

Once more it is difficult to be sure of the precise nature of this criticism. If it means that it does not occur in nature then of course it is false, for we are part of nature and what we do is in *that* sense necessarily natural. If it means that it does not or would not occur in nature without man's intervention then certainly it is true; but by that definition *most* of man's interventions are unnatural, including most medical interventions, and it is difficult to take so broad and unspecific a 'criticism' seriously.

C. TRANS-SPECIES GENETIC MANIPULATION

One of the types of genetic intervention that is regarded as unnatural and therefore morally unacceptable is trans-species genetic manipulation. But apart from a 'gut reaction' that it must be wrong because it is unnatural, what is intrinsically wrong with such genetic manipulation? At its simplest, trans-species genetic manipulation is currently used to create, for example, human insulin for therapeutic use, by transplanting insulin-producing human genetic material into bacteria and then growing the bacteria in bulk and thus producing high quality insulin in bulk. Current research may allow the incorporation of human genetic material into the genome of pigs, which would make their organs less liable to rejection if transplanted into humans. Certainly this is "unnatural" in the sense that such transgenic pigs would not have arisen without man's intervention. But it is difficult to understand what is intrinsically wrong with such interventions, and easy to see, in terms of benefit to mankind, what is potentially good and right about them.

We get closer to a coherent criticism if we understand by "unnatural" something that is "contrary to man's moral nature". But then we need some explanation of why genetic manipulation is "contrary to man's moral nature". *Prima facie*, it seems no more open to such accusations than any other of man's medical activities.

D. A THREAT TO MAN'S MORAL NATURE ?

There is one sense in which genetic manipulation might be foreseen to become contrary to man's moral nature — notably if it destroyed or damaged that moral nature. If one accepts that our moral nature, just like all other aspects of our nature, resides at least in part in our genetic constitution then, in principle, genetic manipulation could be used to destroy, damage, or even merely modify, our moral nature. While such concerns are still in the realms of science fiction, it is as well to confront them before, rather than after, they have become scientifically possible. There might come a time when, for example, a genetic abnormality was discovered to cause an amoral, "psychopathic" type of personality, or an exceptionally violent type of personality. We need to start thinking how we would react to such an admittedly science-fiction-like scenario. Should we allow abortion for such genetic abnormalities, suppose it were possible to discover them by fetal genetic screening? Should we allow experimental gene therapy to replace the abnormal gene for people discovered to have such abnormalities? In the latter case we might well be genetically modifying a person's moral nature by such interventions? Would we necessarily be wrong to try to do so?

E. TOO DANGEROUS A SLIPPERY SLOPE?

A final concern frequently expressed about genetic manipulation, especially if it is done in a way that allows changes to be inherited by subsequent generations, is that it is simply too dangerous. A slippery slope is predicted whereby initially small genetic interventions cause major harms in the future. This is an important moral concern and applies to all new developments. There is always a risk that new developments, even if they are apparently beneficial, may lead to more harm than benefit. The lesson to be drawn from such concerns is not that all new developments must be banned, but rather that they need careful scrutiny. Potential harms need to be anticipated and methods of preventing or minimizing them devised. From that point of view it seems that the introduction of genetic manipulation techniques is being very carefully scrutinized. National committees on genetic therapy have been established with wide representation of expertise and interests. In the U.K. all new genetic therapy has to be scrutinized by such a committee as well as by the existing system of research ethics committees that scrutinize all human medical research projects. In addition, genetic manipulation workers themselves have already widely accepted that their interventions should, to start with at least, be directed at single gene defects that cause serious ill health, and should be limited to somatic cell interventions which would not be inheritable.[23,24] This is not to exclude other developments for all time, but simply to play safe while the new science of molecular genetics is developed.

As Weatherall says "we have no idea how far it will be possible to go in modifying human beings by changing their DNA....It is not possible for one generation to set ethical norms for their great-grandchildren.[14] However as the potential for human molecular biology is so great it is essential that scientists are completely open about their activities and are willing to develop and maintain a continuous debate with the public about the way their field is moving."[25]

While it seems clear, as Weatherall writes, that one society should not set ethical norms for another about how to balance conflicting ethical concerns — respect for autonomy *prima facie* requires respect for differing approaches within a set of common moral commitments — it is also reasonable to argue that certain ethical norms are universal and apply to all societies. Thus, however the balance is set in particular cases and types of cases between the potentially conflicting moral concerns of respect for people's autonomy, beneficence, nonmaleficence, and justice, and a concern for their scope of application; however the balance is set between moral concern for the individual and moral concern for the group; it remains reasonable to argue that these same moral concerns and commitments will and should underlie not only our contemporary assessments of the morality of any new developments in molecular genetics, whether in cancer therapy or any other field of medicine, but also that they will and should underlie the assessments of our successors.[26,27]

REFERENCES

1. **Beauchamp, T. and Childress, J.** *Principles of Biomedical Ethics*, 4th ed.; Oxford University Press: New York, 1994.
2. **Gillon, R.** *Philosophical Medical Ethics*; John Wiley & Sons: Chichester, 1985, and subsequent reprints.
3. **Marie Curie Cancer Care.** *Teaching Ethics — An Initiative in Cancer and Palliative Care*; Marie Curie Cancer Care: London, 1992.
4. **Saunders, D. C., Ed.** *Hospice and Palliative Care — An Interdisciplinary Approach*, 1st ed.; Edward Arnold: London, 1990.
5. **Jeffrey, D. I.** *There Is Nothing More I Can Do. An Introduction to Ethical Issues in Palliative Care*; Patten Press (for Lisa Sainsbury Foundation): Newmill, Penzance, England, 1993.
6. **Kottow, M.** Medical confidentiality: an intransigent and absolute obligation. *J. Med. Ethics* 1986, 12, 117–122.
7. **General Medical Council.** Professional conduct and discipline: fitness to practise; General Medical Council, London.
8. **President's Commission for the Study of Ethical Problems in Medicine and Biomedical and Behavioral Research.** *Screening and Counseling for Genetic Conditions*; U.S. Government Printing Office: Washington, D.C., 1983; pp. 42–47.
9. **Nuffield Council on Bioethics.** *Genetic Screening — Ethical Issues*; Nuffield Council on Bioethics: London, 1993; pp. 41–53 and 65–74.
10. **President's Commission for the Study of Ethical Problems in Medicine and Biomedical and Behavioral Research.** *Screening and Counseling for Genetic Conditions*; U.S. Government Printing Office: Washington, D.C., 1983; pp. 62–63.
11. **Weatherall, D.** Human genetic manipulation. In *Principles of Health Care Ethics*; Gillon, R.; Lloyd, A., Eds.; John Wiley & Sons: Chichester, 1994; pp. 971–983.
12. **Seller, M.** Genetic counselling. In *Principles of Health Care Ethics*; Gillon, R.; Lloyd, A., Eds.; John Wiley & Sons: Chichester, 1994; pp. 961–970.
13. **Thornton, H.** Clinical trials — a brave new partnership? *J. Med. Ethics* 1994, 20, 19–22.

14. **Baum, M.** Clinical trials — a brave new partnership: a response to Mrs. Thornton. *J. Med. Ethics* 1994, 20, 23–25.

15. **Fried, C.** *An Anatomy of Values*; Harvard University Press: Cambridge, 1970, pp.155–182.

16. **Harder, F.** Prophylactic surgery. In *Hereditary Cancer and Preventive Surgery*; Weber, W.; Laffer, U. T.; Durig, M., Eds.; S. Karger: Basel, 1990; pp. 67–69.

17. **Luscher, N. J., Harder, F.** The difficult choice of surgical procedures for breast cancer prophylaxis. In *Hereditary Cancer and Preventive Surgery*; Weber, W.; Laffer, U. T.; Durig, M., Eds.; S. Karger: Basel, 1990; pp. 93–99.

18. **Gillon, R.** *Philosophical Medical Ethics*; John Wiley & Sons: Chichester, 1985, and subsequent reprints; pp. 86–99.

19. **Adelmund, K.** The role of employees. In *The Social Consequences of Genetic Testing*; Rigter, H.; Bletz, J.; Krijnen, A,; Wijnberg, B.; Banta, H., Eds.; Netherlands Scientific Council for Government Policy: The Hague, 1990; pp. 61–64.

20. **Office of Technology Assessment.** *Genetic Monitoring and Screening in the Workplace*; OTA: Washington, D.C., 1990; p. 42.

21. **Nuffield Council on Bioethics.** *Genetic Screening — Ethical Issues*; Nuffield Council on Bioethics: London, 1993; pp. 75–81.

22. **Gillon, R.** Ethical issues in screening for mental handicap. In *Prevention of Mental Handicap: A World View*; Hosking, G.; Murphy, G., Eds.; R. Soc. Med. London, 1987; pp. 35–40.

23. **Committee on the ethics of gene therapy.** Report of the Committee on the Ethics of Gene Therapy, Cmmnd 1788 ed.; HMSO: London, 1992.

24. **Weatherall, D.** *The New Genetics and Clinical Practice*; Oxford University Press: Oxford, 1991.

25. **Beauchamp, T. L.** The 'four principles' approach. In *Principles of Health Care Ethics*; Gillon, R.; Lloyd, A., Eds.; John Wiley & Sons: Chichester, 1994; pp. 3–12.

26. **Gillon, R.** The four principles revisited — a reappraisal. In *Principles of Health Care Ethics*; Gillon, R.; Lloyd, A., Eds.; John Wiley & Sons: Chichester, 1994; pp. 320–333.

Chapter 14

LEGAL ASPECTS

Patrick M. Lynch

CONTENTS

I. INTRODUCTION

Over the past several years dramatic advances have occurred in the molecular genetics of inherited cancer predisposition.[1-6] In addition to shedding important new light on the pathogenesis of common human cancers, these discoveries have provided a novel opportunity to identify individuals who are carriers of deleterious germ-line mutations. With respect to colorectal cancer, the subject of this report, genes responsible for the two leading hereditary disorders have been localized and sequenced. The *APC* gene on chromosome 5q is responsible for familial adenomatous polyposis (FAP).[1-3] At least four genes, members of the mismatch repair pathway, contribute to Hereditary Nonpolyposis

0-8493-4782-3/96/$0.00+$.50
© 1996 by CRC Press Inc.

Colorectal Cancer (HNPCC).[4-7] When appropriate, the *hMSH2, hMLH1, hPMS1,* and *hPMS2* genes will be referred to as the "HNPCC" genes.

Prior to the discovery of the *APC* and HNPCC genes, but accelerated by them, has been an increase in attention devoted to clinical issues in the management of the disorders.[8-11] During this same time period, the relationship between clinicians, family registers, patients, and family members began to show some definition.[12] As in any complex of relationships in modern society, the need began to be appreciated for an ordered set of expectations amongst the members involved in the network. Perhaps more accurately, the lack of existing, well-understood guidelines for exercising rights and responsibilities between groups and individuals left a temporary vacuum.[13-14] The potential for conflict has thus existed between physician and patient, familial disease registers and patients, registers and physicians, patients and their relatives, and patients and health/life insurers. In short, any conceivable relationship has, by its very existence, lent itself to the potential for conflict and the need for conflict avoidance or, failing in that, conflict resolution.

In the pages to follow, areas of potential conflict will be discussed, with attempts made to provide guidance where some consensus exists as to the preventive and remedial measures that might be employed. The setting for this will be the scenario in which a patient with hereditary colorectal cancer interacts with the various groups and individuals who, for better or worse, participate in his or her access to evaluation and treatment.

II. CASE SCENARIO

A 37-year-old woman is seen for her annual gynecologic evaluation by her primary care physician. The physician has just attended a continuing medical education symposium devoted to screening for common malignancies and was struck by a presentation on the potential for genetic testing in families with a strong history of colorectal cancer. He notes in the course of reviewing his patient's medical chart that her father had died of an "abdominal tumor". He then asks the patient if she could elaborate on the information that she has provided years earlier. She reports that indeed her father did have an abdominal tumor at age 43. Although she had been too young to remember any details, she did recall that he had a colostomy for the two years before he died of widespread tumor. When pressed further about the presence or absence of any further family history, the patient reports that indeed there is additional cancer. Her sister, five years older than herself and residing in another city, had recently undergone hysterectomy for a "female cancer". In the course of evaluating her sister, the doctors had found traces of blood in the stool, had done some sort of bowel test and found a small cancer, and removed it at the same time as the hysterectomy. His interest caught by this information, the gynecologist asks if any other, perhaps more remote family members had cancer, particularly on her father's side. She responds that a paternal uncle, still living at age 62, had undergone colon resections for tumor on two different occasions, once at about age 45, and again, more recently.

The patient's physical exam is unremarkable and her blood profile is normal. Before arranging her next annual examination, the gynecologist contacts a general surgeon in the building for advice on whether any further evaluation is warranted. The surgeon recommends contacting the district genetic disease program, which has recently added an adult cancer project and whose director had spoken at the continuing education program that both doctors had attended. The project's director is contacted. On the basis of the information provided, he suggests that two things be done: (1) obtain a gastroenterological consultation, and (2) allow the registry staff to interview the patient further about her family history, document its extent, and verify the information provided so far. The gynecologist makes these recommendations to the patient. She is happy to provide information to the registry although she is concerned that several cousins on her father's side not be contacted as they are members of a religious cult that is opposed to traditional medicine. She also appears somewhat embarrassed about the GI referral but says nothing to the doctor and agrees to the consultation. However, before leaving the office, she tells the scheduling secretary that she hopes the gastroenterologist will not have to do any expensive tests, as she has no insurance and can barely afford her annual primary care visits and Pap smears.

Reluctantly, she sees the gastroenterologist, whose repeat physical exam is normal except for a positive fecal occult blood test, a test which had been negative just the week before. Colonoscopy is recommended and at the time of exam a nearly obstructing mass is found in the descending colon, precluding exam of the proximal colon. Surgery is scheduled.

Meanwhile, the patient has been interviewed by the nurse working for the adult inherited cancer project. Documentation of family history did not demonstrate any additional individuals with cancer, though ancestors of the patient's father could not be traced. Retrieval of hospital records of the father was obtained following submission of a release signed by the patient. Her uncle and sister were contacted by telephone, did confirm their own diagnoses, and also allowed retrieval of their hospital records. This process took six weeks due to the time required for record releases to be sent to the relatives, returned to the registry, forwarded to the appropriate hospitals, and returned with the records. Based on the available information, the director of the registry planned to bring the patient in for counseling in order to communicate the likely presence of HNPCC, based upon the presence of the four individuals with colorectal cancer. Molecular genetic testing would be suggested, specifically the testing of the patient herself via direct mutation analysis, starting with the *hMSH2* gene, followed by linkage analysis if no mutation is identified. Finally, the patient would be urged to consider subtotal colectomy, due to the cancer diagnosed, coupled with the provisional diagnosis of HNPCC. Hysterectomy would also be considered. If a mutation were identified through molecular testing, molecular testing of offspring beginning at about age 18 would be advised, with a recommendation for colonoscopy beginning by age 20-25 in those carrying the same mutation. If no mutations were identified and linkage not informative, similar surveillance would still be recommended, on clinical grounds.

However, by the time documentation of the details of family history were gathered and recommendations formulated, the patient had already undergone surgery, a segmental resection of an invasive adenocarcinoma, with two positive nodes. Adjuvant chemotherapy had already been initiated. Nevertheless, the patient was brought in and the originally planned recommendations provided. Since limited surgery had already been performed, close follow-up was suggested: colonoscopy at six months and endometrial sampling.

Molecular testing was performed and a mutation found in the *hMSH2* gene, obviating the need for linkage analysis. Although her oldest child, a son, was only 12 years old at the time, the patient was anxious to have him tested. The matter remains under discussion. The patient's endometrial and colon cancer-affected sister was also tested and found to be positive for the same mutation. However, she asked that her children, both in their early 20s, not be contacted as they were the members of the religious cult opposed to traditional medicine. The patient's uncle, despite his earlier cooperation in the release of medical information, declined molecular testing and asked that his children not be contacted regarding the evaluation of the family as he did not want them to "worry" about their cancer risk.

The original patient, now six months post-op, was scheduled for follow-up colonoscopy. During the exam, a small mass was identified in the cecum. She is very angry about this finding and, following surgery, prepares to sue all of the doctors involved — the gynecologist, the general surgeon, the gastroenterologist, the medical oncologist, and the registry director, over the costs of the second surgery and the pain and suffering associated with it.

Many legal as well as ethical issues arise in the course of this hypothetical, but quite possible case. These will be discussed in the context of this case, as well as in more general terms. Among the questions to be considered are the following:

1. Is there a relationship between the registry staff, particularly its medical director, and the patient?
2. If so, does this relationship extend to include any of the other family members, most of whom were never encountered in person?
3. If a relationship exists, was there any fault on the part of the registry and its director that would justify their inclusion in a lawsuit against the treating physicians?
4. Was there any negligence on the part of the originally treating gynecologist? The subsequently involved gastroenterologist, surgeon, and medical oncologist? To what standard should they be held?
5. Does it matter in what country these events took place?

6. How should we resolve the matter of the patient's desire to have her son undergo molecular testing?
7. Knowing that the patient's cousins are at 50% risk of HNPCC, does the registry have any responsibility to communicate this risk to them, despite the uncle's and aunt's positions on the matter?

These questions will be taken up individually.

A. RELATIONSHIP BETWEEN REGISTRY AND PATIENT

In the U.S., four elements must be satisfied in order for a patient to successfully bring an action for professional negligence.[15] First, there must be a relationship between the physician (or other professional) and the patient. Second, there must be a breach of this duty (the negligence itself). Third, there must be damage to the patient. Fourth, there must be a cause and effect relationship between the negligence and the damage sustained (proximate causation).

In this case, there is no question as to the existence of a physician-patient relationship regarding the gynecologist, surgeon, gastroenterologist, and medical oncologist. Some question does exist as to the relationship between the patient, registry, and its medical director. One must examine the understanding that would be arrived at by a reasonable patient. This, in turn, depends to some extent on the manner in which the registry was presented to the patient. If it was clearly understood that the family history evaluation was simply a research undertaking with no possible diagnostic or therapeutic implications, then perhaps no relationship exists. If, as in the case here, the registry does undertake to diagnose clinically (via the family history) or on a molecular basis, such a relationship almost certainly does exist. In this case, the impressions of the registry director were communicated directly to the patient. If the registry wished to avoid such entanglements, it might have simply provided an impression to the gynecologist that initially sought advice. Clearly, if the gynecologist assumes the burden of doing all of the communicating with the patient, then the registry will probably be thought of as sufficiently peripheral that no relationship exists. If there is no relationship, there can technically be no negligence, no matter that erroneous or tardy information is provided.

One anticipates that molecular diagnostic laboratories, certainly those operating on a commercial basis, will be held to be as responsible for their results as any clinical laboratory doing routine chemistry and hematology. The more immediate question concerns laboratories that are considered research facilities, but whose descriptions of mutations or carrier status by linkage analysis are relied upon by clinicians in making a genetic diagnosis and offering clinical surveillance and treatment. Among the most important issues is whether informed consent was obtained for the testing and how the terms of the consent are worded.[16-18] Do the clinician and laboratory work together as a team? In the case of the registry medical director and the molecular diagnostics laboratory, the partnership and shared responsibility are evident. Suppose, however, that the gynecologist drew the blood sample in question? Suppose the case involves the physician caring for the patient's uncle or aunt? What risk, if any, is assumed by them for any errors on the part of the laboratory? Conversely, what risk, if any, is shouldered by the registry and laboratory if their (accurate) report is misinterpreted by these same clinicians? Assuming no relationship is held to exist between the laboratory and a given patient, might there at least be a relationship between the laboratory and clinician, such that errors on the part of the laboratory could form the foundation for action by the clinician in the event he or she is sued by the patient?

B. RELATIONSHIP BETWEEN REGISTRY AND RELATIVES

In our example, it is fairly clear that a relationship does exist between the registry and the patient. Does this relationship extend to her sister, uncle, children, and cousins? Unless the relative approaches the registry or the registry approaches the relative and there is mutual, if not formally stated agreement that evaluation will be performed, then no relationship exists. Nevertheless, as in the case of the original patient, even a fairly attenuated involvement could form the basis for an implicit relationship if the individual acts on an implicit recommendation (for testing or clinical evaluation) by the registry and made specifically to that individual, as opposed to a general admonishment to an ill-defined group.

Aside from the question as to the existence of a relationship, can there be found in the law a "duty to warn"?[19,20] As shown below, many if not most genetic counselors feel that such a duty exists, sometimes even if the original patient objects. American case law raises the possibility that such a duty does exist.[21-23] A rather notorious case in California involved a patient who communicated to his psychiatrist an intent to kill his girlfriend.[21] When he carried out this intent, the court found that it was a reasonable that a jury might consider the psychiatrist negligent for failing to notify the party at risk.

C. WAS REGISTRY STAFF AT FAULT IN ANY WAY?

Although the overall scenario described is fairly unusual, it is by no means improbable. Most patients, however aggrieved they may actually be or perceive themselves to be, rarely sue.[24] But when a suit is undertaken, legal representatives of the patient tend to include as defendants any and all individuals and entities that may conceivably be implicated. In this case it is not very surprising that the registry would be included in the action along with the other treating physicians. Given actual knowledge of the increased risk of a second primary cancer of the colon, it might be argued that this should have been passed on to her attending surgeon at an earlier date, along with the recommendation for total colectomy.

One question that exists is the standard to which the registry and its director should be held. Because familial cancer registries are still quite few in number, it would be difficult to find a specific standard to which they should be held.

Because clinical directors may come from many different specialties, a common set of expectations might be difficult to establish. The point being raised here is that although it may not be easy to classify the responsibilities of the registry personnel with any specificity, it is possible that a registry, to the extent it makes any clinical recommendation, may be viewed in the same light as any other clinician, and may not be able to "hide" behind a claim that their efforts were only a research undertaking. Indeed, as cancer genetic services become more "main-stream", as they may be expected to become with the advent of the molecular testing described herein, such litigation may be anticipated to increase.

D. ANY NEGLIGENCE BY TREATING PHYSICIANS?
The various treating physicians and surgeons interacted with the patient in a more traditional, standard fashion. As such, any individual negligence would be measured by existing standards of care. While to some extent such standards have been determined by local patterns of care for similar disease states, in recent years standards for specialists in various fields have come to be regarded in terms of the average practices on the part of clinicians within the same specialty field. As such, the determining issue or question may be: just what should they know about HNPCC and how should their care have been modified? At this writing, HNPCC has been described in all current standard texts on medicine and surgery.[25,26] In specialty areas such as gastroenterology and medical and surgical oncology, it receives considerable attention.[27-29] Consequently, the patient might argue, persuasively, that the doctors should be familiar with the basic principles of its management. Indeed, they did know enough to obtain appropriate consultation and to perform colonoscopic evaluation. However, some consideration should have been given to planned performance of a subtotal colectomy which, despite the absence of compelling data, is generally considered the surgical procedure of choice.[9] At the very least, some attention to pre- or intra-operative evaluation of the right colon could have been given.[30]

III. INTERNATIONAL PERSPECTIVE: VARIATION IN APPROACHES TO COUNSELING

As we have already seen, considerable attention has been devoted to ethical issues in genetic counseling. Applications of ethical principles, and even more so, legal principles, are culture dependent. As such, tremendous variation exists around the world in terms of the approach to genetic counseling. Surveys have been conducted to plumb the nature and extent of these possible differences. Wertz and Fletcher[22] presented clinical case vignettes and sought responses from investigators in 18 countries, most of whom were Western trained and 87% of whom were physicians. The cases had to do with disclosure of test results, disclosure of potentially psychologically distressing information, directive vs. nondirective counseling on reproductive choices, patient privacy vs. relatives' "need to know", and prenatal diagnosis. Broad consensus did exist in most areas. However, disagreement existed in several key areas. One instance dealt with Huntington's disease (HD). A subject with a recent diagnosis of HD refuses to permit disclosure of the diagnosis and related genetic information to siblings at risk. Response ranged from simply protecting the patient's confidentiality, to efforts to persuade the patient to allow release of findings, to providing information (without consent) but limited to directly affecting the relative's risk, to communication of information to the patient's referring physician, thus shifting the burden of decision-making. The competing ethical principles were considered to be patient autonomy/privacy vs. "nonmaleficence" or duty to warn third parties of potential harm. Overall, 58% of respondents (66% outside the U.S.) would warn other family members, despite the breach in confidentiality. A similar difference of opinion existed as to risk of hemophilia A. In HD, only 32% would preserve confidentiality and 10% would allow the patient's own doctor to decide the matter.

In both cases, the competing ethical choices were between autonomy and avoidance of harm. Both dealt with communication of distressing information. One case had to do with ambiguous sex — XY genotype in phenotypic female with infertility, and the other with the carrier status of balanced translocation and risk of Down's syndrome. In the infertility case, 51% (41% outside U.S.) would disclose XY genotype and a similar proportion would communicate translocation carrier status.

Another topic considered was genetic screening and the right of third parties, such as employers, schools, and life and health insurers to receive test results. Consent to release was the main determinant of outcome. If consent was given, 93% would release Huntington's disease results, 89% would release susceptibility to work-related disease to insurers, but only 81% would release the same information to employers. If no consent was given by the patient, only 45% would release the Huntington data, while 40% and 22% would disclose the work-related disease susceptibility to insurers and employers, respectively, without patient consent.

Key issues in the preceding discussion were the identification of areas in which there was a lack of consensus among genetic counselors and the sometimes culture-bound differences that account for the lack of consensus. Because codes of legal conduct broadly follow ethical principles on a country-by-country basis, approaches to counseling and the content of such counseling must be regarded in light of the peculiarities of a given country's history, culture, and religion. Nevertheless, to the extent that a consensus of opinion does exist within a given jurisdiction, that consensus can be viewed as a standard by which the commissions or omissions on the part of an individual practitioner may be judged. Indeed, as the most difficult-to-demonstrate basis for liability is commonly "standard of care", the search for a consensus can become critical in any given case.

IV. DESIRE TO HAVE SON TESTED

The issue of when to test offspring for germ-line mutations predisposing to adult cancer will become a problem in the years to come. Removal of uncertainty may be an important end in itself for many individuals, relieving anxiety about the future even when the results are bad news. Because no clinical evaluation is generally recommended before age 20–25, there is little advantage to testing before this age. Consequently, a policy of refusing to test younger individuals would be reasonable. More problematic is the issue of prenatal testing. Technically, there is no barrier to the performance of amniocentesis for genetic testing in this setting. Certain ethical issues do exist. Because of the incomplete penetrance of mutated mismatch repair genes, malignancy may not occur at all or may not occur until relatively late in life. In addition, the tumors that typically occur are far from lethal, particularly when detected at an early stage. Thus, the impairment can be considered fairly mild or at least preventable.

V. NOTIFICATION OF AT-RISK COLLATERAL RELATIVES

The issue here is confidentiality. The patient's aunt and uncle are both affected with cancer. The aunt carries an *hMSH2* mutation and the uncle is likely to as well, although he refuses testing. For different reasons they refuse to have their children notified of the nature of the problem that exists in the family and the opportunity for molecular testing.

VI. DISCRIMINATION

The health consequences of disease can be distinguished from the economic consequences of being labeled as "diseased", i.e., whether the illness is actually present or whether genetic testing has simply identified risk in an asymptomatic individual. Genetic discrimination has been defined as "discrimination against an individual or against members of that individual's family solely because of real or perceived differences from the normal genome in the genetic constitution of that individual."[31] The fear exists in many individuals with or at risk of hereditary cancer that awareness of their status on the part of employers[32-35] or life and health insurers[36-38] could lead to denial or termination of employment or insurance.

One survey was performed in order to identify actual examples of such discrimination.[38] Cases were solicited from workers in the field of clinical genetics: 29 reports described 41 examples of discrimination, nearly all having to do with employment or insurance. Difficulties included inability to obtain insurance coverage or employment despite evaluations demonstrating physical fitness for the coverage or job involved. Once an individual has health insurance, such as employment-related group coverage, problems of "portability" of the policy to a new job are encountered. This is particularly a problem when one has or may have a "preexisting condition". It is often very difficult for an individual patient to know whether or not their condition is preexisting. The individual is placed, then, in the untenable position of reporting his or her status, without any guidance as to the decision likely to be reached by an insurer, vs. the risk that by failing to report the condition payment will be denied on the basis of falsification of the original application. In such a setting of uncertainty, many subjects are tempted to forego genetic testing for fear that a positive report would be held against them by an insurer or employer.

To date, examples of discrimination have been the exception. The U.S. Congress Office of Technology Assessment (OTA)[39] surveyed leading corporations regarding their employment practices vis-a-vis genetic testing. Of 330 Fortune 500 companies responding, only 20 (6%) utilize any form of genetic screening. Several that had previously utilized such testing have ceased doing so. While it would be important to know the practices of nonresponders to the survey, the prevalence of such testing is undoubtedly low.

The Council on Ethical and Judicial Affairs of the American Medical Association recently expressed its opinion on the matter of genetic testing by employers.[35] It concluded that it would be "generally inappropriate" to exclude from employment those individuals considered to be at increased genetic risk of disease, unless a showing could be made of specific susceptibility to occupational disease. This position is based in part on the typically poor predictive value of genetic testing in terms of the onset, time-course, and severity of disability, due to variable penetrance. Rather, periodic testing of actual fitness for work is advocated.

A task force on genetic information and insurance was formed by the U.S. National Institutes of Health.[40] Its task was to establish the background facts and issues and to formulate recommendations as to how genetic information should be handled in relation to insurance. The effort was carried out in the context of the larger 1994 debate on health care reform in the U.S. and assumed, erroneously, or at least prematurely, that comprehensive reform would occur. Limited to health insurance and not addressing life or disability insurance, the multidisciplinary work-group arrived at the following recommendations: (1) that (genetic) information bearing on health status, past, present, or future, should not serve as a basis for denying coverage or services; (2) health systems should offer universal access to "basic" health services; (3) genetic services should be integrated into the larger system, to include genetic counseling, testing, and treatment for individuals and families; (4) costs of insurance to such individuals and families should not be affected by genetic data; (5) access to services should not depend on employment status; (6) access should depend on an individual's disclosure of genetic information; and (7) pending availability of universal coverage, measures should be taken to reduce discrimination, including a moratorium on the use of testing in underwriting by insurers. It is worth noting that representatives of the American insurance industry withheld their approval from the recommendations provided in the report.

Some remedies against discrimination exist, though their applicability to the specific situation of genetic discrimination remains problematic. In the U.S., the Rehabilitation Act of 1972[41,42] prohibits preemployment inquiry about health or disability, although employment may be conditioned upon passing a medical examination. However, the scope of the law was limited to employers whose work is related to the federal government. The Americans with Disability Act of 1990 broadened the scope of the Rehabilitation Act.[43,44] The legislative history of the Act suggests that "genetic status" was to be within its purview. Whether the Act is actually held to cover genetic discrimination remains to be determined through court proceedings. Unfortunately, in a given circumstance in which discrimination is actually in question, there must be an actual example of discrimination, not the mere fear of it. The burden of proof lies with the complaining, would-be employee. The Act specifically does not prohibit insurers or other health-benefit administrators from underwriting and classifying risks, presumably including genetic risks.[44] This raises the much larger issues having to do with allocation of costs of treating individuals with such "preexisting" conditions as hereditary risk. It may be less expensive in the long run to perform molecular testing on those at risk of inherited colorectal cancer and it may be cheaper to carry out periodic surveillance in those carriers of susceptibility than it would be to treat advance disease. Nevertheless, from the standpoint of insurers, either preventive measures or treatment of late disease will be more expensive than would be coverage of an individual truly at "average" risk of colorectal cancer. If coverage of individuals with increased susceptibility is offered at the same price as that for the general population, then the increased cost of their coverage will be shifted to those at average risk. In short, fair treatment is not necessarily the same as equal treatment.

In countries with universal health coverage, a greater emphasis exists on preventive measures. Because all diagnostic, treatment, and prevention costs are distributed widely over society, systematic savings due to prevention programs carry great appeal. By the same token, however, rationing of services must occur throughout the health care system. Under these circumstances the question may be: is it cheaper to identify individuals at risk of HNPCC and carry out surveillance colonoscopy than it is to simply treat cancer when it occurs?

There has been established an Ethical, Legal, and Social Issues (ELSI) working group within the Human Genome Initiative at the U.S. National Institutes of Health and the Department of Energy.[40] Projects carried out under the auspices of ELSI have begun to provide guidance for the genetic testing of susceptibility to such diseases as cystic fibrosis (CF). Specifically, concerns about informed consent to testing, appropriate education of individuals, families at risk, and health-care providers have been addressed.

Because of the recent isolation of HNPCC and familial breast cancer (*BRCA* 1 and 2) genes, ELSI and cooperating agencies have undertaken sponsorship of projects addressing psychosocial issues in familial breast and colorectal cancer, excluding FAP. These include preparedness to undergo molecular genetic testing. One of ELSI's goals was to organize the participating institutions into a consortium that would be able to collectively address certain issues of common concern.

In early 1995, investigators from the 11 projects met with ELSI officials and other interested parties, consultants, and observers. Three of the projects deal with colorectal cancer. Concerns were repeatedly raised regarding the adequacy of the process by which the studies were introduced to the prospective subjects or participants and informed consent obtained.

Experience gained from cystic fibrosis research raised specific issues of risks associated with genetic testing, including the following:[45]

1. Risk of losing insurance
2. Risk of losing employment
3. Stress imposed on interpersonal relationships
4. Risk to self esteem
5. Revelation of nonpaternity

The opinion that such risks should be communicated to study participants was strongly held by the ELSI staff, although many project directors expressed concern that raising such issues might unduly frighten prospective study participants.

In communicating possible study benefits to would-be participants, the informed consent process was thought to benefit from the inclusion of the following disclosures:

1. Molecular genetic testing is not perfectly predictive — existing tests fail to detect mutations in as many as 20–40% of individuals who appear to have "typical" HNPCC. Moreover, the determination that one carries a mutation simply indicates a *susceptibility* to the disease. This is known because about 20% of carriers never develop cancer or do so very late in life, due to reduced penetrance of the gene mutation.
2. Absence of mutation does not mean that cancer will *not* occur, since noncarriers have the same cancer risk as the rest of the population. In Western countries such risk may be relatively high, as much as a 6% lifetime risk.
3. There is no proof that identification of carrier status will lead to interven-

tions that improve longevity. While colonoscopy for detection of early polyps (adenomas) and cancer are *believed* to be beneficial, there exists no proof to date that this is the case.

4. While relief of uncertainty as to carrier status may be beneficial both for carriers and noncarriers alike, there again is no proof that for any particular individual this will be the case.

Recognizing the considerable limitations that exist in our ability to communicate accurate risks and benefits of molecular genetic testing, it is important to stress that the acquisition of such knowledge is precisely the objective of the projects being conducted.

VII. "MARKETING" OF MOLECULAR GENETIC TESTING

A variety of questions pertain to the question of public interest in molecular genetic testing. How will physician providers and at-risk subjects alike view the availability of molecular testing for colorectal cancer? What will be the range of tolerance of imperfection in predictive potential of HNPCC testing? Are there issues unrelated to molecular testing itself that bear on an individual's interest in testing? Several speakers addressed these issues. Dr. Neil Holzman of Johns Hopkins University spoke to the need for "marketing research", identifying just who will use genetic testing and what barriers may prevent its use.[46] In order to answer this question, greater understanding of the real and perceived risks and benefits must be achieved. Examples from cystic fibrosis, Down's syndrome, and Huntington's disease were cited for the proposition that different people react differently to testing, depending on the anticipated level of certainty regarding test outcome and severity of disease.

Preliminary information was presented on these issues, based on discussions with members of consumer "focus groups".[47] Participation was solicited through newspaper advertisements and respondents were divided into those with and at-risk of breast cancer, men from families with breast cancer, and average risk population. Various socioeconomic strata (SES) were represented. Higher SES groups were most interested in issues of test cost, accuracy, and availability of further information upon which to make decisions. Lower SES consumers were more likely to harbor misconceptions, such as the notions that particles in the air increased risk. They were more interested, for example, in whether test results would be helpful to their children and whether testing would need to be repeated. Recommendations for content of explanations to consumers in anticipation of testing included: correction of misconceptions about disease and testing, the meaning of test results whether positive or negative, advantages and disadvantages of follow-up diagnostic and therapeutic measures, and clarification of risks associated with disclosure of information to third parties.

VIII. CONCLUSION

Legal considerations in the provision of family history evaluation have been shown to be rather complex. In the setting of a poor outcome or unfulfilled expectation, the patient and members of his or her family may be viewed by the defensive clinician as adversaries, interested only in reaping a financial windfall or injuring a professional reputation. Of course there will always be the possibility of a "worst-case" scenario, as described at the outset. Yet from the standpoint of professional negligence, we are simply applying well-accepted legal principles to the newly evolving field of clinical cancer genetics.

Distinct from relational problems between the patient and clinician or registry are insurance and employment difficulties that may plague individual patients. These difficulties vary considerably from country to country.

In the future, evolution and clarification of standards of practice in the field of clinical cancer genetics will certainly occur. Situations will continue to exist in which clinical research overlaps with or spills over into clinical practice. Here, establishment of boundaries will be necessary in order that patients, as research participants, may better understand the nature of their relationship with their health care provider/clinical investigator. Indeed, as the source of data characterizing risk of genetically determined cancer shifts from research laboratories to clinical service laboratories, so too will patients, providers, and laboratory directors themselves need to determine whether different standards and expectations do exist.

REFERENCES

1. **Bodmer, W. F., Bailey, C. J., Bodmer, J., et al.** Localisation of the gene for familial adenomatous polyposis on chromosome 5. *Nature (London)* 328: 614–616, 1987.
2. **Kinzler, K. W., Nilbert, M. C., Su, N. L.-K., et al.** Identification of FAP locus genes from chromosome 5q21. Science 253: 661–665, 1991.
3. **Spirio, L., Olschwang, S., Groden, J., et al.** Alleles of the APC gene: an attenuated form of familial polyposis. *Cell*, 75: 951–7, 1993.
4. **Peltomaki, P., Aaltonen, L. A., Sistonen, P., et al.** Genetic mapping of a locus predisposing to human colorectal cancer. *Science* 290: 610–612, 1993.
5. **Lindblom, A., Tannergard, P., Werelius, B., and Nordenskjold, M.** Genetic mapping of a second locus predisposing to hereditary non-polyposis colon cancer. *Nat. Genet.* 5: 279–82, 1993.
6. **Aaltonen, L. A., Peltomaki, P., Leach, F. S., et al.** Clues to the pathogenesis of colorectal cancer. *Science* 260: 812–16, 1993.
7. **Nicolaides, N. C., Papadopoulos, N., Liu, B., et al.** Mutations of two PMS homologues in hereditary nonpolyposis colon cancer. *Nature (London)* 371: 75–80, 1994.

8. **Lynch, H. T., Smyrk, T. C., Watson, P., et al.** Genetics, natural history, tumor spectrum, and pathology of hereditary nonpolyposis colorectal cancer: an updated review. *Gastro* 104: 1535–49, 1993.

9. **Fitzgibbons, R. J., Jr., Lynch, H. T., Stanislav, G. V., et al.** Recognition and treatment of patients with hereditary non-polyposis colon cancer (Lynch syndromes I and II). *Ann. Surg.* 206: 289–95, 1987.

10. **Houlston, R. S., Murday, V., Harocopos, C., Williams, C. B., and Slack, J.** Screening and genetic counselling for relatives of patients with colorectal cancer in a family cancer clinic. *Br. Med. J.*, 301: 366–8, 1990.

11. **Vasen, H. F., Mecklin, J.-P., Watson, P., et al.** Surveillance in hereditary nonpolyposis colorectal cancer. An international cooperative study of 165 families. *Dis. Colon Rect.*, 36: 1–4, 1993.

12. **Lynch, P. M. and Winn, R. J.** Clinical management of hereditary nonpolyposis colon cancer. High-risk clinics and registries. *Hematol. Oncol. Clin. N. Am.*, 3: 75–86, 1989.

13. **Lynch, P. M. and Lynch, H. T.** Medical-legal aspects of familial cancer. *J. Leg. Med.* 4: 10–16, 1976.

14. **Lynch, P. M.** Jurisprudential considerations in the evaluation and screening of high-risk patients. *Front. Gastrointest. Res.* 10: 55–63, 1986.

15. **Reilly, P.** Genetic counseling and the law. In P. Reilly: *Genetics, Law and Social Policy.* Harvard University Press, Cambridge, pp151–89, 1977.

16. **Rosoff, A. J.** Informed Consent: A Guide for Health Care Providers. Aspen, Rockville, Md., 1981.

17. **Elias, S. and Annas, G. J.** Generic consent for genetic screening. *N. Eng. J. Med.*, 330: 1611–13, 1994.

18. Office for Protection from Research Risks (OPRR): *Protecting Human Research Subjects: Institutional Review Board Guidebook.* U.S. Department Health Hum Svc, Pub Health Svc, NIH, Ofc of Extramural Res, U.S. Government Printing Office, Washington, D.C., 1993.

19. **Geller, G., Tambor, E. S., Bernhardt, B. A., et al.** Physicians' attitudes toward disclosure of genetic information to third parties. *J. Law Med. Ethics* 21:238–40, 1993.

20. **Pelias, M. Z.** Duty to disclose in medical genetics: a legal perspective. *Am. J. Med. Genet.* 39: 347–54, 1991.

21. Tarasoff v. Regents of the University of California. 131 Cal. Rptr. 14, 1976.

22. **Wertz, D. and Fletcher, J. C.** *Ethics and Human Genetics: A Cross Cultural Perspective.* Springer-Verlag, New York, pp536, 1989.

23. **Andrews, L. B.** Legal aspects of genetic information. *Yale J. Biol. Med.* 64: 29–40, 1991.

24. **Huycke, L. I. and Huycke, M. M.** Characteristics of potential plaintiffs in malpractice litigation. *Ann. Intern. Med.* 120: 792–8, 1994.

25. **Mayer, R. J.** Tumors of the large and small intestine. In Wilson, J. D., et al. (Eds.): *Harrison's Principles of Internal Medicine*, 12th ed,, McGraw-Hill, New York, pp1289–1295, 1991.

26. **Kodner, I. J., Fry, R. D., and Birnbaum, E. H.** Colon, rectum, and anus. In Schwartz, S. I., et al. (Eds.) *Principles of Surgery*, 6th ed., McGraw-Hill, New York, pp1191–1306, 1994.

27. **Bresalier, R. S. and Kim, Y. S.** Malignant neoplasms of the large and small intestine. In Sleisenger, M. H. and Fordtran, J. S. (Eds.) *Gastrointestinal Disease* (4th ed.), W.B. Saunders, Philadelphia, 1989.

28. **Olabaster, O.** Colorectal cancer: epidemiology, risks, and prevention. In Ahlgren, J. D. and Macdonald, J. S. (Eds.) *Gastrointestinal Oncology*, Lippincott, Philadelphia, pp 243–259, 1992.

29. **Cohen, A. M., Minsky, B. D., and Schilsky, R. L.** Colon cancer. In DeVita, V. T., Hellman, S,. and Rosenberg, S. A., (Eds.), *Cancer: Principles and Practice of Oncology*, 4th ed., Lippincott, Philadelphia, pp929–77, 1993.

30. **Winawer, S. J., Enker, W. E., and Levin, B.** Colorectal cancer. In Winawer, S. J. (Ed.) *Management of Gastrointestinal Diseases,* Gower Medical, New York, pp 27.1–27.40, 1992.

31. **Natowicz, M. R., Alper, J. K., and Alper, J. S.** Genetic discrimination and the law. *Am. J. Hum. Genet.* 50: 465–475, 1992.

32. **Canter, E. F.** Employment discrimination implications of genetic screening in the workplace under Title VII and the Rehabilitation Act. *Am. J. Law Med.* 10: 323–47, 1984.

33. **Gostin, L.** Genetic discrimination: the use of genetically based diagnostic and prognostic tests by employers and insurers. *Am. J. Law Med.* 17: 109–35, 1991.

34. **Andrews, L. B. and Jaeger, A. S.** Confidentiality of genetic information in the workplace. *Am. J. Law Med.* 17: 75–108, 1991.

35. **Orentlicher, D.** (Council on Ethical and Judicial Affairs, Am. Med. Ass'n.): Council report. Use of genetic testing by employers. *JAMA,* 266: 1827–30, 1991.

36. **Jecker, N. S.** Genetic testing and the social responsibility of private health insurance companies. *J. Law Med. Ethics* 21: 109–16, 1993.

37. **Ostrer, H., Allen, W., Crandall, L. A., et al.** Insurance and genetic testing: where are we now? *Am. J. Hum. Genet.* 52: 565–77, 1993.

38. **Billings, P. R., Kohn, M. A., de Cuevas, M., et al.** Discrimination as a consequence of genetic testing. *Am. J. Hum. Genet.* 50: 476–82, 1992.

39. Office of Technology Assessment, U.S. Congress: *Medical testing and health insurance,* US Government Printing Office, Washington, D.C., (OTA-H-384., 1988.

40. Task Force on Genetic Information and Insurance (NIH/DOE Working group on Ethical, Legal, and Social Implications (ELSI) of Human Genome Research, U.S. Government Printing Office, Washington, D.C., 1993.

41. 29 U.S. Code, Sec. 701–796, 1982.

42. **Canter, E. F.** Employment discrimination implications of genetic screening in the workplace under Title VII and the Rehabilitation Act. *Am. J. Law Med.* 10: 323–47, 1984.

43. 42 U.S. Code 12111-12201, 1990.

44. **Maffeo, P. A.** Making non-discriminatory fitness-for-duty decisions about persons with disabilities under the Rehabilitation Act and the Americans with Disabilities Act. *Am. J. Law Med.* 16: 279–326, 1990.

45. **Clayton, E. W.,** personal communication.

46. **Holzman, N.,** personal communication.

47. **Geller, G.,** personal communication.

Chapter 15

THE CANCER FAMILY STUDY UNIT

Brian K. Hart, Maria Shaffer-Gordon, and John J. Mulvihill

CONTENTS

I. INTRODUCTION

A. PREVIEW

The findings summarized in this volume and elsewhere[1-5] resulted from the effort of many individuals, often reporting on the experience or interdisciplinary research with a few as one or as many as several dozens of families with an apparent excess of cancer. The experience and research findings emerge from the interaction of family members with various clinicians and other staff

0-8493-4782-3/96/$0.00+$.50
© 1996 by CRC Press Inc.

members who act on the behalf and authority of a clinical director or principal investigator.

This chapter focuses on those staff members and workers whose functions can be subsumed in the title, the Cancer Family Study Unit. These personnel are often invisible, sometimes receiving credit in publications, sometimes not. Their activities are articulated in few places,[6,7] perhaps most often in applications for research funds from granting agencies. That description, which may make the difference in a grant award, is confidential and unavailable to teams that aspire to address local concerns and research opportunities involving cancer families.

Dr. Henry T. Lynch's Hereditary Cancer Institute and its affiliates at Creighton University, Omaha, NB have been described.[8] Anne Krush, the long-term head of family study logistics at Creighton, went on to perform a similar function for families with colorectal cancer ascertained at the Johns Hopkins Hospital. She has coauthored the most definitive and recent description of family studies units.[7] Blattner set down the strategy and structure of the productive family studies unit at the U.S. National Cancer Institute, launched in 1962 by Miller and Fraumeni, and continued serially by Li, Mulvihill, Blattner, Tucker, Parry, and others.[6]

The family studies approach to understanding human disease, of course, is neither confined to studies of cancer nor to the United States.[2,4] As a classic means to dissect out environmental and genetic determinants of disease, the required resources have been widely mobilized, as seen in the body of literature on familial aggregation, ecogenetics, and the like.[5,9]

We present a view of the crucial elements for a successful cancer family studies unit. It is based on 20 years of experience with cancer family studies at the U.S. National Cancer Institute leavened with family studies research for cancer and other diseases in a U.S. research university, the University of Pittsburgh. An exact and universal formula is impossible, in part because of differences in culture, resources, and space. However, the most important determinant of the make-up and work of a cancer family studies unit is its purpose and mission.

B. PURPOSE OF THE UNIT: RESEARCH OR SERVICE?

Most units serve a supportive function. They have no purpose of their own, but are the vital infrastructure to accomplish a main goal in the most economical and efficient way possible. In their daily work, the unit's staff members perceive that their role is to perform a service. The clinical or scientific leader of the unit must decide whether the overall mission is to address clinical service needs or to serve a research purpose. The unit functions differently, depending on the primary goal.

A cancer family study unit focused on *research* has rigid protocols that set down in great detail the required tasks, policies, and procedures. The function may be limited to a specific epidemiologic study design with, for example, questionnaires that are highly computer-compatible, using only close-ended queries, and giving little latitude for probing or eliciting information. Exactly the same questions are asked, in person, by telephone, or in writing, in exactly the same way to avoid bias introduced by an interviewer. Only specific tumor types, certain age groups, or distinct geographic regions may be eligible for inclusion. Answering a specific research question in a timely and definitive way is the purpose. Often, the goal is not to benefit individual families or persons because the study results are handled statistically and reported in the aggregate. Continuity or ease of follow-up is not an issue.

On the other hand, when the mission of the cancer family study unit is *service* to a clinical institution or to individual persons and families, the function is much different. Policies and procedures, although very clear, are more a set of general guidelines than a rigid prescription. Priority is given to offering feedback to study subjects and referring physicians, even if definitive results are not available. Long-term contact and rapport are important, and slavish attention to every last form might be secondary.

Of course, the mission of a cancer family studies unit may require a blend of the two purposes. This dual objective may compromise achievement of either goal, but may be necessary for reasons of funding and responsiveness to the public.

Once the overall mission or purpose is decided, the unit can be developed and families can be contacted (Figure 1). In consultation with statisticians and potential laboratory collaborators, specific protocols, procedures, and policies should be determined. Questionnaires, forms, and databases have to be designed, perhaps by modifying existing resources to serve the local purpose. Since most units have some research mission, an early step is to seek the approval of the local institutional review board. This crucial step, often requiring four months' time, has to be done with an eye toward the approvals that might be needed by collaborators in diverse parts of the world, where standards and expectations might differ from the local culture. Likewise, most external funding agencies also demand approval by a local institutional review board. As discussed below, the U.S. National Institutes of Health has issued guidelines[10] that go beyond consideration of physical risk to address the specific hazards of family studies including possible coercion to participate, psychological risk, invasion of privacy, breach of confidentiality, and loss of insurability.

Cancer family studies are labor intensive and, in most organizations, new personnel must be hired for the specialized purpose. New funds will be needed for office and shipping supplies, computers, files, travel, and operating costs. Obviously, external funds are available more easily for addressing a specific research question than for clinical service purposes. In the current U.S. health care system, the specialized services of a cancer family study unit are not likely to be paid for unless an actual outpatient consultation is done by a physician. If blood, endoscopic, or imaging tests are recommended to at-risk persons,

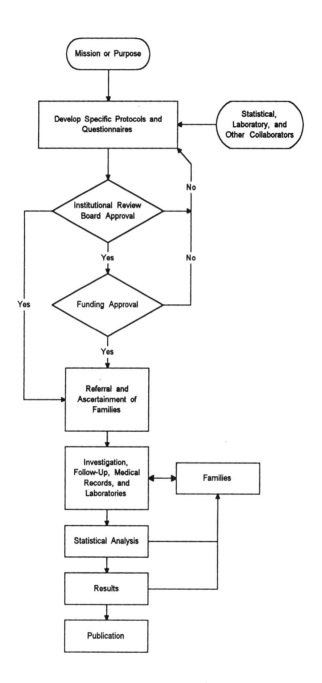

FIGURE 1. The family studies process.

charges may be denied because they are for screening currently healthy persons. Review of submissions for funding and institutional review board approval may well demand revision of protocols and questionnaires.

II. EVALUATING A FAMILY

Perhaps the best way to describe the functions of a cancer family study unit is to follow a typical sequence of tasks in the interactions with a single family: ascertainment, pedigree development, record collection, hand and electronic filing and data management, and collection of biological specimens, sometimes by means of field trips.

A. ASCERTAINMENT

If segregation analysis is a goal of the research design, strict rules for ascertainment and documentation of how and from what source families are ascertained is necessary. Otherwise, there may be many routes for locating families. The proband, or index patient, is the individual whose diagnosis brings the family to the unit's attention. Potential probands may be identified by collaborating physicians, especially practicing oncologists. A letter to medical oncologists, radiotherapists, and oncologic surgeons is another good ascertainment source. The physician may contact his or her patients directly or may give the family studies unit permission to contact them. Other sources of probands include reviews of hospital records, and state or local tumor registries. Health and welfare organizations, local or national cancer information services, and genetic counseling centers can be made aware of a study; they may give their clients information about how to contact the family study unit or may ask for an individual's permission to be contacted. The medical or lay literature could reveal families whose original investigators might be willing to facilitate recontact. Lay support groups may also be a good source of referrals. An exhibit or poster in a medical meeting, hospital, or health fair might lead some families to refer themselves. Self referral often occurs after research findings are publicized in the popular media. Finally, current participants in a study may know of families similar to theirs.

The Office for the Protection from Research Risk (OPRR) of the U.S. National Institutes of Health issues guidelines for human studies research.[10] A principal ethical concern is that probands and families should not be unduly persuaded to participate in research. Lay support organizations may exert such influence. Patients may feel that their care under a private physician may be compromised if they refuse to participate or refuse referral.

Once the proband has agreed to participate in the study, attempts are made to recruit other members of the family. There are different ways to accomplish this, each of which poses potential ethical problems discussed in the OPRR Guidelines.[10] When the proband is the family recruiter, relatives will be insulated from pressure from investigators, but may be subjected to extra pressure from the proband who might have a personal interest in seeing that the research is completed. Alternatively, the proband may be unwilling to recruit other family members to avoid revealing that he or she has the disease of interest. The recruitment of family members directly by the investigator may be considered an invasion of privacy by some relatives.

The approach chosen must be tailored to each family to maximize privacy and confidentiality and minimize the disruption of the family dynamics and the pressure exerted on family members to participate. It is generally advisable to have one family member talk with another to ask if the investigator may contact him or her. The family studies team must not reveal personal or medical information about one family member to another unless the first person has given permission to do so.

Despite the potential pitfalls in enrollment, it is gratifying that so many people are, in fact, willing to participate in cancer family studies. These families have personal experience with cancer, usually in more than one close relative, and appreciate medical and research attention to the family's problem — especially if the research is geared toward the early detection, treatment, and prevention of cancer. Relatives often participate with the expectation that even if the research does not directly benefit them, it may benefit other members of their families.

B. DEVELOPING THE PEDIGREE

The pedigree is the most essential information in any family study. The research team should pick a standard manner in which to record pedigrees, such as the one set by the *American Journal of Medical Genetics*.[11] A template can be used to draw squares and circles by hand, or a computer program such as Cyrillic[12] or Pedigree/Draw[13] can be used. It is helpful to mark on the pedigree which family members have been examined by investigators, which have donated specimens, and whether a diagnosis of cancer has been verified by medical records or is based solely on the report of the proband or another family member. All types of cancer in family members should be recorded, not just the particular cancer of interest. The age at diagnosis, examination, or death may be noted, along with relevant exposure history or other pertinent information.

Each individual in the pedigree should have a unique identification number. The Family Studies Unit of the U.S. National Cancer Institute uses an identification number composed of a four-digit family number (assigned consecutively in time), a two-digit generation number, and a three-digit number for each member of that generation. Rather than numbering generations sequentially, the proband's generation is assigned "01", the preceding generations are given odd numbers, and the subsequent generations are given even ones. This allows for continuation of the pedigree to future and past generations without the need for renumbering every time a generation is added.

The initial pedigree may be drawn based on interviewing the proband and other relatives, or it may be based on one or more questionnaires. The accuracy of the pedigree should be verified by cross-checking with other informants, being careful not to break confidences. Every family seems to have its own medical genealogist. It is neither sexist nor "ageist" to state that, in our experience, an elderly woman is often the best source of information. Informants may give contradictory information, which the researchers must try to resolve, e.g., with medical records or death certificates. The pedigree will need to be revised and updated as more information is obtained from family members and medical records and as time passes. All pedigrees and paper notes should be dated. Computerized pedigrees require less time to update.

Information concerning the presence or absence of cancer should be collected on at least the proband's parents, brothers, sisters, and children (first degree relatives) and aunts, uncles, grandparents, and grandchildren (second degree relatives). If other, more distant relatives are thought to have had cancer, they, along with the intervening relatives, should be noted on the pedigree. A pedigree with three generations is more likely to provide information on the possible mode of transmission than a nuclear family pedigree, especially if cancer or susceptibility to cancer is transmitted in an autosomal dominant or X-linked recessive manner. One also needs to determine whether parents of an affected individual were blood relatives or may have been members of a relatively small, possibly inbred population, as consanguinity increases the chance of detecting an autosomal recessive pattern of inheritance. The family's ethnic origins should also be noted.

As the pedigree is extended, relatives with an increased risk to develop a specific type of cancer may be identified. Members of the family study unit may be able to assess what family members understand about the types of cancer in their family. Even before exact risks are known, relatives can be given information about early signs of cancer and available tests to detect cancer at an early stage when it is likely to be curable. Unit staff can answer questions and dispel myths, such as that cancer is found only in family members of one sex or relatives with a certain eye color. From their contacts with various agencies and organizations, members of the family study unit may suggest medical and social resources and literature that could be beneficial to families.

Although the report of a family member is good evidence that cancer has occurred,[14] medical records are needed for validation, especially if research is the unit's mission. Sometimes, cancer patients themselves poorly understand or communicate their own medical histories. In extended families, the validity of a reported cancer decreases as degree of relationship increases. Medical records resolve inaccuracies or confusion and may reveal the exact histopathologic diagnosis. Besides paper records, pathology specimens (slides and blocks) may be useful as described later; such specimens are requested in the same manner as paper records.

When family members have been seen in the investigator's own facility, the documentation is complete and easy to obtain. Usually, affected individuals in a family have used many institutions and clinicians in more than one geographic area. Much detective work may be required to locate records. The requirement to obtain a signed release form from each subject further complicates the process. To avoid long delays in obtaining the needed information, the family studies team must:

- Decide exactly what information is deemed essential;
- Carefully identify the facilities most likely to have the essential records; and,
- Obtain releases containing sufficient identifying information: full name at that time, dates of birth, treatment, or examination, the specific reason for the request, investigator's name and address, and signature of subject or guardian, or if the subject is dead, next-of-kin. If the subject is dead, the facility may require a copy of the signatory's power-of-attorney or other documentation showing proof that he or she is next-of-kin.

Death certificates may be useful when medical records are unavailable, but caution is necessary in making interpretations from them. Cancer may have been present but not listed or insufficiently described, especially if it had been successfully treated. For example, the researcher may be interested in insulinoma and the death certificate may simply state "pancreatic cancer" or "abdominal carcinomatosis." Conversely, if the cancer is difficult to diagnose or is rapidly fatal, it might not have been recognized until autopsy. The validity of death certificate information varies with tumor type, year of death, geographic region, death in hospital or elsewhere, autopsy status, etc.[15] The information on death records must be viewed in light of the statements of family historians or of information in other medical records.

In the U.S., access to death records varies from state to state. In many states, copies of records may be obtained by anyone. In other states, death records are protected documents and must be requested either in a manner similar to obtaining medical records or upon approval of a research protocol. Internationally, laws protecting privacy rights and use of protected data in medical research will need to be investigated early in the study to avoid delays in obtaining information later. The National Center for Health Statistics of the U.S. Department of Health and Human Services publishes a useful booklet of the names and addresses of state vital records agencies.[16] Fees for vital records may be expected.

C. DEVELOPING THE QUESTIONNAIRE

Questionnaires are used to obtain genealogical and medical information. The content and form of questionnaires vary, depending on whether an interviewer or the subject will complete them. In either case, the investigator must avoid ambiguous or unfocused questions.

Questionnaires designed to be completed by the subject have additional requirements. Instructions for completing a questionnaire should be clear and easily understood, even by an individual whose education is limited. It must be assumed that the person completing the questionnaire does not have much medical knowledge. The readability of the questionnaire is greatly improved when it is brief and contains few big words. Plenty of white space surrounding questions will benefit those with reduced visual acuity. The typeface chosen should be no smaller than standard typewriter pica.

All questionnaires should request identifying information (name, address, telephone number, sex, date of birth, race, and Social Security number in the U.S.). Extra space should be included for responses that do not fit in the space provided and for additional information that the subject feels is important. Completion improves when short responses are expected. Whenever possible, responses should be circled words ("yes", "no", or "don't know") or checked boxes. This strategy limits the variability of responses and aids in data entry and analysis.

No questionnaire is perfect: all should be pretested by representatives of the target group. Once a study is underway, revisions should be kept to an absolute minimum, but emerging information may mandate a change in questions.

A family history questionnaire lists an individual's parents, siblings, grand-parents, and other relatives who have had cancer. Information on children, aunts, uncles, nieces, and nephews may also be collected. There should be enough room to write names, addresses, and dates of birth and death. Additional questions may be asked of all family members or only of those with cancer. A proxy or surrogate may be necessary if an affected person is unavailable, incompetent, or deceased. Concerning each cancer, appropriate questions include the type and primary site, and when and where the diagnosis was made. There should be space to list more than one cancer. The exact questions depend on the types of cancer being studied and the known or potential risk factors. A questionnaire might generate new hypotheses as well as attempt to test current ones. Questions about noncancerous conditions, all surgeries, and medications taken during the individual's lifetime may be asked. Lifestyle questions, including those about smoking history, alcohol consumption, occupational exposures, and nutrition are often desirable, but can add undue length for the quality and utility of the information. The informant may be asked what he or she believes is the cause of cancer in the family. For practical, as well as ethical, reasons, the questionnaire should seek only the most necessary information. An early version of the National Cancer Institute questionnaire has been published.[17]

As with all research and clinical issues, compliance with the questionnaire is variable. Questionnaires mailed "cold" to prospective subjects often have the lowest compliance rate. Compliance is better when the subject completes the questionnaire in the study office site and best when an interviewer helps to complete the questionnaire. The complexity of the questionnaire and design of the study often determine which method of completion is used.

D. FILES

Because each family study is different, there is no ideal way to record and organize data; however, some general recommendations can be made. A separate master log book to index all families in the study should be maintained. At minimum, this log should include the surname of the proband and a unique identification number. The date and source of referral and ascertainment, hospital record number of the proband, and other brief comments, such as the diagnosis, may also be included.

Specific information on any individual in a family should be stored in a separate folder labeled with the family's identification number and some further system of numbering or lettering for the individual. The types of information frequently found in a folder include a working copy of the pedigree, a face sheet, questionnaires, consent forms, records release forms, results of examinations, results of tests performed during the study, copies of previous medical records or death certificates, and records of contacts. Medical records include pathology, surgery, diagnostic imaging, and laboratory reports. If the study is being done in a hospital using only patients who have been seen at that hospital, then the clinical records may be filed elsewhere. Contact records include written correspondence and notes concerning interviews and phone calls, field trips, etc. Copies of form letters may be kept, or a log sheet for form letters may be used instead. A running log sheet can be useful to include dates when questionnaires and consents were sent and received, when records and pathology specimens were requested and received, when records and specimens were reviewed by a staff member, types of surgery including when and where performed, and types of treatments given and reasons for treatment. Paper files are inevitable in family studies, but electronic files are far preferable for consistency and ease of use in data analysis. Computerized data are essential for identifying the mode of inheritance (segregation analysis), for determining the location of a gene associated with a cancer of interest in one or more families (genetic linkage analysis), and for genetic epidemiology. The family studies database is much different from a clinical database because it must show relationships of family members. The questionnaire always dictates the design of the database. A database that bears no resemblance whatever to the questionnaire will be difficult and costly to use.

A useful database design for the small family studies unit is a system called the Genetic Epidemiology Management System (GEMS).[18] This model consists of a family studies database core that can be used as is or with extensions. The model is a relational database formed from interlocking data tables containing various aspects of the family file. These tables include, but are not limited to, data pertaining to the family, individual personal data, medical history, diagnostic test data, and laboratory data. The database mirrors closely in electronic form the paper files discussed above. In addition, pedigree and genetic marker data can be stored along with demographic data and medical history.

Of course, the particular database application platform will vary according to the available resources and data manager's preferences. The prime determinants of the database are the intended use and the likely users. Considerations in choosing a database application are size and geographic scope of the study; ease in developing the database, data entry, and obtaining data reports; and available funding. As more powerful computers become available for less cost, more powerful off-the-shelf database application programs are developed that will easily meet most specifications. In a family study of abdominal aortic aneurysms,[19] one author is using Borland* Paradox* for Windows™** to develop a full-featured family studies database for a large number of families.

Further considerations in choosing a database application are

- Will the application manage all of the data in each of the needed tables?
- Is the application capable of managing a large relational database? Some applications claim this capability, but the size of the database may be limited.
- Will the application run at reasonable speed on the available equipment and within budget limitations? It is much less expensive to run an application on a personal computer, but will this serve the needs of all the users?
- If a local or wide area network is in use, will the application run successfully in that environment? While some database applications will run on a network, they may not be suited for multiple users.
- Will the application allow for relatively easy retrieval of data in a format required by analytical software?
- How will data be protected? Too often, carefully maintained paper files exist in a poorly developed electronic format that is readily available to anyone. Identifiable data must be protected from scrutiny in electronic form as well as in paper form.

In general, data must be backed up regularly to avoid loss. Sufficient staff support must be available to ensure timely data entry, verification, and updates. Good planning will save considerable analysis time and protect against security breaches and data loss.

E. SPECIMENS

The types of specimens collected in a family study depend on the study's purpose. Specimens that are frequently collected include blood and tumor and normal tissue for cytogenetic studies (analysis of chromosome number and structure), loss of genetic heterozygosity (loss of variation at a specific genetic locus), loss of genetic imprinting (loss of differential expression of genes,

---

* Borland and Paradox are registered trademarks of Borland, Inc.
** Windows is a trademark of Microsoft Corporation.

depending on transmission from mother or father), oncogene activation (at what level is an oncogene being transcribed), genetic linkage analysis, and biomarkers of tumors or exposure to potential carcinogens. Laboratory collaborators should be consulted for specific requirements involving sample type, size, and methods for shipping and handling beyond what is shown in Table 1.

Tumor tissue may become available for research when a participant undergoes surgery or when the next-of-kin permits an expeditiously performed autopsy. The surgeon, operating room nurse, pathologist, or pathology technician should be given a specific protocol to follow ahead of time. The desire of the participant to proceed with the research should be stressed to the primary physician. Tissue should be obtained from the original site and from metastases. Specimens should be viable (non-necrotic) true tumor, not from the margin, with as little normal tissue as possible. Many tumors have a low proliferative index, which necessitates cell culture. If there is extensive necrosis or microbial contamination, the sample will not grow.

TABLE 1
Methods for Transporting Specimens

Type of Specimen	Purpose	Method of Transport	Viability Limit
Solid tissue[a]	Cytogenetics	In tube with culture medium, room temperature, next day air	24 hours
Solid tissue[a]	Loss of heterozygosity	In container without medium, frozen, on dry ice,[b] next day air	As long as is frozen
Solid tissue[a]	Oncogene expression[c]	In container without medium, frozen, on dry ice,[b] next day air	As long as is frozen
Slide or tissue block	Pathology	Room temperature	Indefinite
Blood	Cytogenetics	In heparin tube, room temperature, next day air	24 hours
Blood	Genotyping for linkage analysis	In EDTA tube, room temperature, next day air	3–4 days[d]
Blood	Loss of heterozygosity	In EDTA tube, room temperature, next day air	3–4 days[d]
Serum	Tumor markers, other analyses	Plastic tube with screw top, frozen, dry ice[b] or wet ice or refrigerant gel pack, next day air	As long as is frozen. If cold, depends on tests to be performed.
Other	Various	Depends on sample	Depends on sample

[a] Solid tissue may be tumor or normal tissue.
[b] Approximately 10 pounds of dry ice is necessary to ensure that sample stays frozen during transit. Dry ice is considered to be a hazardous material, and appropriate labeling is required. The contents of the box should also be listed.
[c] Must be frozen immediately in liquid nitrogen.
[d] Delays in processing may reduce usable DNA yields.

Tissue samples should be handled sterilely. The surgeon may be able to set aside a sterile sample for research in the operating room, or the pathologist can cut the sections needed under sterile conditions. In most hospitals, the pathologist controls the sample and his or her cooperation is crucial. A person present in the operating room, such as a circulating nurse, can also be helpful.

Enough tumor tissue to establish a cell line should be obtained. If there is extra tissue, direct karyotyping (chromosome analysis) without cell culture may be possible. The larger the sample, the more culturing techniques the laboratory can employ to increase the chance of successful culture, and some may be cryopreserved as a backup in case of culture failure. Karyotyping may identify areas of the genome associated with transformation, metastasis, etc. Numeric or structural aberrations may suggest locations of oncogenes or tumor suppressor genes. Normal DNA could be extracted from peripheral blood lymphocytes, normal tissue from the affected organ, or skin taken from a punch biopsy or the edge of a surgical incision.

Tumor and normal tissue to be used for cytogenetic studies should be transported in media or buffered saline in a sterile container. The containers holding the tissue specimens should be filled to the top with culture medium so that the tissue does not dry out during transport.

Samples of fresh, unfixed, sterile tumor and normal tissue are also needed for studies of loss of heterozygosity and imprinting and for oncogene activation. Solid tissue samples for these studies should be frozen at low temperatures as quickly as possible. For studies of oncogene expression, samples must be frozen immediately in liquid nitrogen to prevent degradation of RNA; this is generally hard to accomplish unless the surgeon is committed to the research study. Additional pieces of tumor, fixed for the preparation of paraffin tissue blocks and for electron microscopy, may also be desired.

Whole blood samples may be used for cytogenetic analysis and molecular studies such as linkage analysis and loss of heterozygosity and imprinting. It may be desirable to immortalize lymphocytes as a source of normal DNA for future use. Recent transfusions of whole blood may affect the results of these studies. Generally, the accepted practice is to avoid drawing blood samples for 120 days after a whole blood transfusion. Blood may certainly be drawn earlier after packed red cell transfusions unless the research protocol includes erythrocyte typing. Serum samples may be used to develop nongenetic methods for early detection of cancer, e.g., tumor markers, or for microbial serology, carcinogen detection, etc.

All tubes should be labeled with the participant's name and specimen type (primary tumor, metastasis, normal tissue, skin, blood, etc.). Different types of tissue must be sent in separate containers to prevent confusion and to maintain the correct temperature.

If there is advance notice, it is best to send the proper containers for specimens, boxes for mailing, airbills, and other labels to the hospital ahead of time so that no time is wasted in searching for these items when it is time to collect and ship. If a member of the family study unit is not able to go to the hospital to pick up the samples, the assistance of a family member may be helpful.

Noninfectious blood samples are not considered hazardous material by the U.S. Postal Service and major express carriers. They should be transported in a container designed to hold vials of blood. The container should include or be surrounded by absorbent material such as paper toweling and be sealed in a leakproof plastic bag. These should be placed in an outer container which will not break during transport, such as a corrugated cardboard box.

International shipments require declaration forms in order to be cleared by customs officials. The declaration form must specifically state the contents of the package and its purpose. Noninfectious human blood is easily received and is usually not delayed unless it is improperly identified. An important precaution is to identify the sample as human and for diagnostic or research purposes. It is also helpful to include a letter signed by the principal investigator attesting that the sample is noninfectious. With unusual or infectious specimens, it is advisable to consult with the carrier, the appropriate customs service, and in the U.S., the Office of Health and Safety of the Centers for Disease Control in Atlanta, Georgia.

It is best to avoid sending or receiving samples on a weekend. The best time to send specimens is on a Monday, Tuesday, or Wednesday to maximize the possibility that laboratory personnel will be available to process the samples immediately. The laboratories need sufficient notice to prepare for arrival of specimens and have a technician available for immediate processing. If the specimen must arrive on a weekend or holiday, special arrangements may have to be made.

In some cases, it may be wise to choose a collaborator in the participant's area or to pay a local laboratory to process or analyze samples rather than trying to transport them to one's own laboratory and taking the risk that they may be unusable.

In addition to fresh specimens, it may be useful to obtain old paraffin-fixed or frozen pathology specimens. This resource is of particular value when the subject is deceased and blood or fresh tissue specimens are unavailable. Slides and tissue blocks are kept for varying lengths of time, depending on the hospital. Tissue section slides can be used to confirm a diagnosis of cancer, especially if no pathology records are available. Although cytogenetic studies of fixed specimens are not possible, DNA can be extracted from them. Polymerase chain reaction techniques can be used to amplify DNA for genotyping.

Depending on the exact protocol and tumor types under investigation, there may be a need to collect other specimens such as urine, stool, semen, breast fluid aspirates, and cytologic samples from cervix, lung, colon, bladder, etc.

F. FIELD TRIPS

On occasion, a field trip may be necessary, perhaps more often when the primary purpose of the family study unit is for research rather than for service.

Justifications for a field trip may be urgency, ease of access, saving of expense, and certainty of proper procedures. A key family member may be scheduled for surgery and local personnel cannot be mobilized for the correct collection of operative and other specimens. A relative may be near death and finally willing to donate blood for research purposes. A disabled patient might not be able to travel from home. The team may wish to assess the local environment and to rapidly collect information and blood from a large kindred at a family reunion assembled for the unit's convenience and to increase participation. It might be good to involve local clinicians in the investigation to benefit from their rapport and promote further cooperation. It may be less expensive to send one or two researchers out, rather than to bring a number of family members in to the medical center. If clinical evaluations and specimen procurement are done by the family study unit, they have no one to fault but themselves if anything goes wrong, such as obtaining blood in the wrong type of tube.

Of course, travel can be expensive, especially if flying is required. Field situations are not familiar and may lack facilities for required examinations or specimen procurement. Emergency medical backup is uncertain. Issues of privacy, confidentiality, coercion to participate, and even personal liability may arise. The bulk of transporting supplies needed for safely collecting specimens (and disposing of sharps, etc.) can be inconvenient and even prohibitive.

If a field trip is ever envisioned, it should be planned for ahead of time, before the need suddenly arises on a Friday afternoon. Transportation and local arrangements are unforeseeable, but the inventory of provisions should be planned out, even to the point of having an emergency travel bag always at hand. Such supplies may be paper (a working pedigree, questionnaires, consents, records release forms, mailing envelopes, packaging supplies) and other materials, such as blood collection supplies, local anesthetic, transport media, sharps containers, and so forth, as dictated by the protocol and the experience in one's own unit. If a purpose of a field trip is to see large numbers of subjects, then a package of forms, labels, tubes, etc. for each person is assembled and a detailed timetable of events is prepared with assignments for each team member. A critical list has telephone numbers for family members, collaborating laboratories, and even airlines. Another occasionally valuable document is an official letter from a senior administrator who explains and authorizes, for example, the transport of blood and of intravenous equipment, for inspectors and customs officials.

To provide for both the family's and the team's convenience, field trips can be made to a cooperating physician's office, a public place such as church hall or a private home. A local family member may be willing to accompany the family study unit members and introduce them to their relatives. A letter stating the purpose and objectives of the trip should be mailed to those whose participation is desired. Although an advantage of the field trip is the ability to explain the nature and purpose of the study to everyone at once, knowing in advance what will be expected will place the participants at greater ease and improve the quality and timeliness of informed consent.

The ethical considerations described earlier for ascertainment of subjects and collection of family data must be more carefully considered when a field trip is to be made. Relatives may be more reluctant to decline to participate when the rest of the family is present and when one or more family members have a personal stake in the outcome of a study. The confidentiality of subjects may be compromised if the interviews are conducted during the field trip: the disease status of an affected family member could become common knowledge, despite his or her wishes. Field trips are an extremely useful tool for the family study unit, but this convenience must not be allowed to override the subject's right to provide informed consent and to privacy, even within the family structure.

III. RESOURCES

A. STAFF

The purpose of a family studies unit will determine the staff required. A clinically oriented unit will need the skills of a physician, nurse, social worker, and genetic counselor. A research-oriented unit will need the talents of a genetic epidemiologist, computer systems analyst, and data clerks. However, in either case, the staff must be competent to handle confidential research records, patient contacts, and/or biological specimens. The unit's staff must have good interviewing skills, basic biomedical vocabulary, and be able to make interpretations from verbal histories and medical and vital records. A basic knowledge of genetics and cancer, including laboratory procedures, is also useful.

In either type of unit, the staff must have very good organizational skills. Juggling telephone calls, appointments, follow-up letters, release forms, biological specimen collections and the like for an entire family or many families are time-consuming tasks. Good clerical support will allow the professionals to spend more time with the tasks that only they can do. Other support services include phlebotomy and specimen transport logistics. A local resource, such as a clinical research center, may be employed for these tasks.

Predicting the number of staff needed is difficult. The extent of pedigree development differs widely from one study to another. For example, one study may focus on first degree relatives only, while another expands each family to third degree relatives. The number, length, and type of interviews and follow-up interviews must be considered. No one is school-trained to staff a cancer family study unit. Genetic counselors and nurses are excellent leaders, especially when service is the prime mission. A nurse, especially an oncology nurse, comes with all the jargon and awareness of cancer treatment. A genetic counselor is especially qualified to explain the results of genetic studies to the subjects. Both nurses and genetic counselors can be extremely useful in developing the questionnaire, interpreting medical data, and in making referrals when outside services are indicated. The general skills that can be honed on the job are sensitivity to a range of anxious people and scrupulous attention to detail coupled with the ability to dart from task to task.

B. SPACE

Space considerations for the family studies core are, of course, driven by the amount of staff support required. Other considerations, though, will increase the initial space estimates. A family studies unit requires file space, supply cabinets, and perhaps refrigerators and freezers. The average family file size can easily exceed the size of an average hospital chart, depending on the number of family members and the types of records maintained. Beyond ordinary office supplies, the unit must have the needed venipuncture and specimen collection materials, blood tubes, mailing kits, overnight mail supplies, and forms. Consideration must be given to the confidentiality due subjects when assigning space.

C. HARDWARE

The requirements for computer hardware are largely dependent on the database software. In a large family study, a local area network is a minimum recommendation. As all the family studies staff will need access to the database regularly, a multiuser environment will protect data security and allow for easy maintenance. In a very small family study, a single personal computer may be sufficient. Certainly where possible, faster computers will free the staff from long waiting periods to access and process data.

Further considerations for the family studies office are necessary. Photocopiers and laser printers should be available so that material presented to patients and their families has a professional appearance. Documents need to be printed on a variety of formats: plain paper, envelopes, labels, and letterhead paper. A large office can be hampered by having a single laser printer with only a letter-sized paper tray. The essential telefacsimile machine should be a dedicated unit because confidential documents are sent and received.

Each staff member needs a seperate telephone line. Modem lines should be separate from the voice telephone lines so that study subjects can always get through. An answering machine or voice mail is important so that participants or their physicians can leave messages at any time. Accepting collect calls or providing toll-free incoming call service will improve subject compliance.

D. SOFTWARE

The choice of software will be driven by the choice of computer hardware. Both will be subject to the preferences of the users and the personnel setting up the system. New, more powerful products appear on the market at a frenetic pace, so it is impossible to recommend specific software products.

The core package will be the database management program, software that is crucial for the efficiency of the entire study. The database must handle large amounts of data and be easy to use, protected from unauthorized use, and reliable. What one investigator uses and prefers for personal contacts or for office records will seldom meet the needs of the family studies unit. In a large clinical family studies unit, highly specialized software that is not commercially available may be needed. In unusual circumstances, very specialized software may need to be written. In a small center, however, commercial packages can be used to develop a relational family studies database that will run on a specific computer.

Although important, database software is not the only package required for family studies. Family studies units contact many subjects, schedule appointments, and produce large quantities of mail. A full-featured word processing program capable of merging personal information files with form letters is indispensable. Contact management software is very helpful with managing appointments, keeping track of meetings, etc. This type of software, as with the others, is available for network use. When used, it is possible for one member to schedule meetings, fields trips, and patient contacts involving more than one member of the team without needing to speak with everyone involved.

Pedigree drawing and pedigree management software can extend the usefulness of the hand-drawn version immensely. Current versions of such software allow the team to maintain in a single pedigree file much of the information found on several family studies forms. As a bonus, they can produce presentation-quality drawings. Cyrillic[11] allows for the storage, display, and basic analysis of genetic marker data, and is straightforward to use. It can produce data files ready for analysis by several well-known genetic analysis programs.

Analysis software is usually used at several points in a family study. To test for modes of inheritance, segregation analysis software, such as SAGE,[20] PAP,[21] FISHER,[22] and POINTER[23] is needed. Software for linkage analysis includes LIPED,[24] LINKAGE,[25] MENDEL,[22] and with limits, Cyrillic.[11] Segregation analysis and linkage analysis software are often obtained together in package form, as with MENDEL and FISHER. These programs, with other related software, form part of the dGene software package.[22]

Data analysis is seldom limited to genetic analyses and environment certainly plays a role in the development of cancer. Statistical software to analyze host characteristics and environmental risk factors for cancer include SAS[26] and SPSS,[27] two widely used statistical packages. These programs can be used to calculate risk, incidence, and other useful statistics.

One other consideration in planning for software is portability of data. Word processing software may be capable of creating and mantaining a database, but it would be foolish to keep duplicate files of names and addresses for producing mail merge files: the needed data will already be maintained in the database. We recommend using a single hardware platform for as many applications as possible. The choice of IBM* and IBM-compatible, Apple Macintosh™**, or other platforms is the prerogative of the individual family studies unit; any will capably handle the workload. Choosing software that can transfer data among application programs will save frustration and lost time in the future.

Conversely, genetic analysis software, although available for personal computers, will run much faster on a RISC processor-based workstation such as those available from Hewlett-Packard, Sun Microsystems, and other companies. Genetic analyses are much more computation-intensive than many other types of analysis, requiring a great deal of computer processor time to complete. The data for these analyses must be generated on the desktop computer and moved to the workstation. Having network connections or modem links eliminates the need for reentering data and reduces errors.

IV. INTERDISCIPLINARY ASPECTS

A. COLLABORATORS

Family studies are interdisciplinary in nature and typically require a variety of laboratory investigators, including cytogeneticists, molecular geneticists, clinical chemists, pathologists, immunologists, and cell biologists. Laboratory investigators advise on the crucial design of a study and on the practical details of obtaining specimens, i.e., how much material is needed, how samples should be handled and transported, etc. Frank discussions and brief memoranda are needed to clarify each investigator's role in the project and rights to data and credit.

B. RELEASE OF RESULTS

Investigations may have clinical or research purposes, frequently both. Results may be used for diagnosis and for identification of high-risk family members. Tests done primarily for research purposes may yield information that is useful for the participant's medical care. Other results are uninterpretable until an entire family study is completed or additional families have been studied. Hence, it is best to have outlined the plan for dissemination of results to study participants, their clinicians, collaborators, and the scientific community before any data are collected.

Patients should be apprised of the results of standard clinical laboratory tests such as hematologic and chemistry values. The release of research tests depends on prior agreement with the subject. Some results (e.g., presence of a certain antibody, HLA typing) are exploratory investigations that have a scientific rationale but cannot be interpreted until additional studies are done or follow-up conducted.

If information from laboratory tests performed for research purposes is to

---

* IBM is a registered trademark of International Business Machines Corporation.
** Apple is a registered trademark and Macintosh is a trademark of Apple Computer, Inc.

be shared with a personal physician, the subject must agree to this release of information. If tests were done for research purposes, the results need not be relayed to a physician, since the clinical interpretation of such results is problematic. Release of results to collaborators depends on prior agreements within the team. There is likely a core group that needs access to all data and collaborating investigators who need to correlate their data with the pedigree, clinical diagnoses, age, sex, etc., but not necessarily with results of other laboratories. Authorship credit is controversial and rules are changing. Nonetheless, it is better to be inclusive rather than exclusive about authorship, as long as authors assume the primary responsibilities that journal editors impose. Even collaborators who are acknowledged should agree to such credit. Family members sometimes appreciate a reprint of a publication that is largely based on their family.

As outlined in the report of the Task Force on Genetic Information and Insurance,[28] the development of tests that predict an individual's likelihood to develop a particular disease carries with it the possibility of genetic discrimination along with the potential benefit of developing preventive strategies. The availability of information concerning genetic risk could jeopardize a person's access to life insurance, health care coverage, or treatment for a condition because it was deemed to be "preexisting" and therefore excluded from coverage. Genetic discrimination for employment and insurance has been documented for genetic diseases other than cancer.[29] Participants in family studies should be made aware of these potential problems.

Individuals who participate in family studies of cancer should be given the opportunity to refuse to receive test results that would reveal their likelihood to develop cancer. The one possible exception to the "right not to know" would be if early treatment of a genetic disease might improve the individual's prognosis. The results of laboratory research tests should be communicated to participants by a qualified family study unit member, preferably a nurse, genetic counselor, or physician. As much time as necessary should be taken to make sure that the participant comprehends the results. With the participant's permission, it may be important to contact other relatives, advise them of their risk, and offer appropriate testing.

ACKNOWLEDGMENTS

The authors would like to thank Robert E. Ferrell, Ph.D., Susanne Gollin, Ph.D., Christopher Aston, Ph.D., and Lisa Parker, Ph.D. for their contributions to this chapter and their invaluable assistance to those involved in family studies at the University of Pittsburgh, and to Pamela St. Jean, Ph.D. for her helpful criticism. Mr. Hart expresses his thanks to Robert E. Ferrell, Ph.D. for providing him the opportunity to employ his otherwise-learned skills within the area of family studies and to Pamela St. Jean, Ph.D. who so gracefully helped him to refine them. Ms. Shaffer-Gordon likewise expresses thanks to

Michael B. Gorin, M.D., Ph.D. Dr. Mulvihill takes this opportunity to thank the many unsung family studies research assistants that he has had the pleasure of working with directly (in reverse chronological order, as memory permits): Carina Rodriguez, Maria Shaffer-Gordon, Sadie Holmes, Melissa Berry, Carolyn Collins, Sharon Doyle, Nancy Ebby, Andy Shafear, and Terry Duel.

This work is supported in part by the following grants: American Cancer Society Grant EDT-80 (The Ecogenetics of Pancreatic Cancer: A National Registry of Families); National Heart, Lung, and Blood Institute Grant 5RO1HL444682 (Genetic Basis of Abdominal Aortic Aneurysm); and Pennsylvania Lions Sight Conservation and Eye Research Grant (Genetics of Age-Related Maculopathy).

REFERENCES

1. **Mulvihill, J. J., Miller, R. W., and Fraumeni, J. F., Jr.,** Eds., *Genetics of Human Cancer*, Raven Press, New York, 1977, 519 pp.
2. **Müller, H. J. and Weber, W., Eds.,** *Familial Cancer*, S. Karger, Basel, 1985, 292 pp.
3. **Lynch, H. T. and Hirayama, T.,** *Genetic Epidemiology of Cancer*, CRC Press, Boca Raton, FL, 1989, 361 pp.
4. **Phillipe, P.,** *Les Familles à Cancer*, Éditions MALOINE, Paris, 1989, 228 pp.
5. **King, R. A., Rotter, J. I., and Motulsky, A. G., Eds.,** *The Genetic Basis of Common Disease*, Oxford University Press, New York, 1992, 978 pp.
6. **Blattner, W. A.,** Family studies: the interdisciplinary approach, in Mulvihill, J. J., Miller, R. W., Fraumeni, J. F., Jr., Eds., *Genetics of Human Cancer*, Raven Press, New York, 1977, 269.
7. **Krush, A. J. and Evans, K. A.,** *Family Studies in Genetic Disorders*, Charles C Thomas, Springfield, IL, 1984, 239 pp.
8. **Lynch, H. T., Fitzsimmons, M. L., Lynch, J. F., and Watson, P.,** A hereditary cancer consultation clinic, *Neb. Med. J.*, 74, 1989, 351.
9. **Khoury, M. J., Beaty, T. H., and Cohen, B. H.,** *Fundamentals of Genetic Epidemiology*, Oxford University Press, Oxford, 1993, 383 pp.
10. **U.S. Department of Health and Human Services,** Public Health Service, National Institutes of Health, Office of Extramural Research, Office for Protection from Research Risks, *Protecting Human Research Subjects: Institutional Review Board Guidebook,* U.S. Government Printing Office, Washington, D.C., 1993, 5–42.
11. **Anon.,** Instructions for contributors, *Am. J. Med. Genet.,* 49, 142, 1994.
12. **Chapman, C. J.,** A visual interface to computer programs for linkage analysis, *Am. J. Med. Genet.*, 36, 155, 1990.
13. **Mamelka, P. M., Dyke, B., and MacCluer, J. W.,** *Pedigree/Draw for the Apple Macintosh:* Population Genetics Laboratory Technical Report No. 1, Southwest Foundation for Biomedical Research, San Antonio, Texas, 1993, 81 pp.
14. **Love, R. R., Evans, A. M., and Josten, D. M.,** The accuracy of patient reports of a family history of cancer, *J. Chron. Dis.*, 38, 289, 1985.
15. **Percy, C. P., Stanek, E., III, and Gloeckler, L.,** Accuracy of cancer death certificates and its effect on cancer mortality statistics, *Am. J. Public Health*, 71, 242, 1981.

16. **National Center for Health Statistics,** Where to Write for Vital Records, U.S. Department of Health and Human Services, Public Health Service, Centers for Disease Control, DHHS Publication Number (PHS) 90–1142, Atlanta, GA, 1990.

17. **Anon.,** Appendix, *Genetics of Human Cancer,* Mulvihill, J. J., Miller, R. W., and Fraumeni, J. F., Jr., Eds., Raven Press, New York, 1977.

18. **Kompanek, A. J., Kauffman, E. R., Blaschak, J., and Chakravarti, A.,** GEMS: a comprehensive database for genetic epidemiological studies, *Am. J. Hum. Genet.,* 51, A153, 1992.

19. **Majumder, P. P., St. Jean, P. L., Ferrell, R. E., Webster, M. W., and Steed, D. L.,** On the inheritance of abdominal aortic aneurysm, *Am. J. Hum. Genet.,* 48, 164, 1991.

20. S. A. G. E.: *Statistical Analysis for Genetic Epidemiology,* Release 2.1, Department of Biometry and Genetics, LSU Medical Center, New Orleans, 1992.

21. **Hasstedt, S. J.,** *Pedigree Analysis Package,* version 3.0, Department of Human Genetics, University of Utah, Salt Lake City, 1989.

22. **Lange, K., Weeks, D., and Boehnke, M.,** Programs for pedigree analysis: Mendel, Fisher, and dGene, *Genet. Epidemiol.,* 5, 471, 1988.

23. **Lalouel, J. M. and Morton, N. E.,** Complex segregation analysis with pointers, *Hum. Hered.,* 31, 312, 1981.

24. **Ott, J.,** A computer program for linkage analysis of general human pedigrees, *Am. J. Hum. Genet.,* 28, 528, 1976.

25. **Lathrop, G. M., Lalouel, J. M., Julier, C., and Ott, J.,** Strategies for multilocus linkage analysis in humans, *Proc. Natl. Acad. Sci. U.S.A.,* 81, 3443, 1984.

26. **SAS Institute, Inc.,** *SAS/STAT® user's guide,* release 6.03 edition, SAS Institute, Inc., Cary, NC, 1988, 1028 pp.

27. **SPSS, Inc.,** *SPSS/x User's Guide,* Release 3.0, SPSS Inc., Chicago, 1988, 1072 pp.

28. **NIH-DOE Working Group on Ethical, Legal, and Social Implications of Human Genome Research,** *Genetic information and health insurance,* National Institutes of Health, National Center for Human Genome Research, NIH Publication No. 93-3686, Washington, D.C., 1993, 32 pp.

29. **Billings, P. R., Kohn, M. A., de Cuevas, M., Beckwith, J., Alper, J. S., and Natowicz, M. R.,** Discrimination as a consequence of genetic testing, *Am. J. Hum. Genet.,* 50, 476, 1992.

Chapter 16

THE HEREDITARY
CANCER PREVENTION SERVICE

Ophira Ginsburg and Steven A. Narod

CONTENTS

I. INTRODUCTION

Recent advances in the fields of clinical and experimental cancer genetics have prompted several academic and private centers in North America to set up familial cancer assessment services for high-risk individuals. These centers are designed to offer comprehensive risk assessment, to recommend screening protocols and to arrange for appropriate referrals. The McGill University Hereditary Cancer Prevention Service is designed to integrate genetic counseling and molecular diagnostic testing for members of families with dominant cancer syndromes.

Cancer families may be identified through many different sources. An astute physician may recognize that there are too many cancers in a family to be explained by chance, and that hereditary predisposition seems to be a more likely explanation. Unfortunately, not all cancer patients are asked about their family history, and many clinicians are unaware of all of the relevant familial cancer patterns. The members of the families themselves may feel that they are genetically predisposed and might seek counselling directly. Often these families are prompted by a particular media event which draws attention to one of the hereditary aspects of cancer.

In some situations, hospital registries may be used to identify individuals who are most likely to carry a susceptibility gene. These patients may have cancer at a site which is commonly hereditary — examples include retinoblastoma, medullary cancer of the thyroid, and pheochromocytoma. They may be recognized because of an unusually early age of onset of cancer; for instance, breast cancer appearing in a woman in her thirties or premenopausal endometrial cancer signal the possibility of genetic predisposition. Women with multiple primary cancers of the ovary and breast, or of the colon and endometrium, may belong to families with the breast-ovarian cancer syndrome or hereditary non-polyposis colon cancer (HNPCC), respectively.

Another source of referral may be other cancer researchers. In the course of a case-control study, or a follow-up study, a colleague in a department of epidemiology may have asked detailed questions about family history of his study subjects. Those subjects who respond positively are potentially members of cancer families. These subjects may be sources of cancer families, provided that appropriate steps are taken to ensure confidentiality, that permission is obtained from the treating physician, and that the patients are given the opportunity to refuse participation prior to being contacted by the geneticist.

Each of these methods has been a source of cancer families in the McGill Cancer Family Clinic. However, we also were interested in answering the fundamental question "Should every patient with cancer have a family history taken?" and in estimating the yield of such a comprehensive approach. To answer this question, we distributed a questionnaire to all cancer patients attending any of several outpatient cancer clinics at two of the teaching hospitals affiliated with McGill University. This questionnaire was originally created at the suggestion of physicians in the Department of Immunology as a means of obtaining relevant family information for those patients who were referred for screening tests, including CA-125 and prostate specific antigen. If these individuals reported multiple affected family members, they were routinely referred to the Division of Medical Genetics for additional investigation. It was later felt that it would be useful to distribute the same questionnaire to cancer patients attending outpatient clinics in an attempt to estimate the frequency of hereditary cancer syndromes among the patients followed at McGill University. For comparability, the same questionnaire was distributed to unselected patients in the outpatient departments of the Division of Immunology. The questionnaire is distributed and collected by the clinic personnel and is self administered.

II. QUESTIONNAIRE FOR HEREDITARY CANCER PREVENTION SERVICE

Certain forms of cancer run in families. This questionnaire asks about your family history in order to see if there may be a pattern of cancer in your family. We hope this will be valuable in preventing future cases of cancer. This questionnaire is voluntary and all information is confidential. We may contact you by telephone regarding this information.

Name_____   Today's Date_____

Address _____

Telephone: home _____   work: _____

Have you previously been diagnosed with cancer? _____ Yes _____ No

    If yes, type _____   At what age _____

    Physician _____   Hospital _____

FAMILY HISTORY

	Breast Cancer	Colon Cancer	Ovarian Cancer	Other (specify)
Mother	_____	_____	_____	_____
Father	_____	_____	_____	_____
Sister(s)	_____	_____	_____	_____
Brother(s)	_____	_____	_____	_____
Children	_____	_____	_____	_____

MOTHER'S SIDE

Aunt(s)	_____	_____	_____	_____
Uncle(s)	_____	_____	_____	_____
Cousin(s)	_____	_____	_____	_____
Grandmother	_____	_____	_____	_____
Grandfather	_____	_____	_____	_____

FATHER'S SIDE

Aunt(s)	_____	_____	_____	_____
Uncle(s)	_____	_____	_____	_____
Cousin(s)	_____	_____	_____	_____
Grandmother	_____	_____	_____	_____
Grandfather	_____	_____	_____	_____

NOTE: If more than one relative has been diagnosed with cancer please indicate number of persons on the line.

III. THE EVALUATION PROCESS

This questionnaire was first distributed in October 1991. We have now collected and processed 411 questionnaires from cancer patients, and 317 questionnaires from a sample of patients with other medical conditions. The questionnaire also carries the comment that the patient may be contacted by telephone by members of the Division of Medical Genetics. The family history is divided into paternal and maternal sides in order to more efficiently separate the nonhereditary from the possibly hereditary forms.

Completed questionnaires are reviewed by one of the genetic counselors and are evaluated for a possible genetic component. In the first step, the forms are separated into the categories nonhereditary and possibly hereditary. The assumption is made that if there are few, or no cancers reported among the first and second-degree relatives, then it is unlikely that a more detailed inquiry will reveal a significant pattern of cancer susceptibility. The patients who are judged to be nonhereditary at this step are sent a form letter indicating this assessment.

The remaining forms (possibly hereditary) undergo a second level of evaluation. The patients are telephoned by a genetic counselor or genetic counseling student. A complete pedigree is taken over the telephone. This includes information on the site and age at diagnosis of cancers in all first- and second-degree relatives. Questions are also asked about bilaterality and the presence of multiple primary cancers. Pedigrees are extended as far as possible in order to include as many affected relatives as are known to the proband. If it is clear at this stage that the case does not qualify as a hereditary cancer family syndrome, the patient is told this over the telephone. However, all patients are encouraged to recontact the genetics service should new cases of cancer be identified in the family. These patients are also sent a letter. Based on our experience, it is sufficient that the genetic counselor completes the second evaluation alone.

The completed pedigrees are reviewed by the cancer genetics team, which includes two counselors and a clinical cancer geneticist, in order to attempt to distinguish between likely and unlikely examples of hereditary cancer syndromes. After discussion, those individuals thought to belong to cancer families are telephoned a second time and are invited to attend an in-person genetic counseling session. The session begins with a review of the patient and family history, with clarification and supplementation of exisiting information. The proband will be asked to obtain additional key information, such as ages at diagnosis of cancer in relatives or the confirmation of a primary site. They may be asked to contact specific relatives who hold key information or to provide consent to review medical records. The counselor will respond to questions posed by the relatives, who are invited by the proband to telephone the genetics service themselves if they wish. However, at no time will the genetics service directly contact a family member for information; all such requests are directed through a family member who has already made contact with the service.

The patient is given a detailed evaluation and risk assessment. The fundamentals of genetics are discussed, including the genetic basis of disease and the principles of gene transmission, penetrance, sporadic cases, etc. The different options for screening are then discussed. Relatives who are also eligible for screening are described in general terms. The discussion of screening tests may include the benefits and limitations of mammograms, physical examinations, ovarian and endometrial ultrasound, and endometrial biopsy. In selected high-risk cases the advantages and disadvantages of screening vs. prophylactic surgery are also discussed. Other areas of cancer prevention are raised to the extent to which knowledge is available. These include dietary recommendations and the known risks and benefits associated with the use of oral contraceptives and hormonal replacement therapy. Women considered to be at high risk for breast cancer are informed of the tamoxifen cancer prevention trial and are given the telephone number of the coordinators of local study centers.

In some cases of known autosomal dominant cancer syndromes, it may be possible to offer molecular diagnosis. These DNA tests either involve linkage analysis, or direct sequencing of cancer genes for mutations. Linkage analysis is offered to families with the breast-ovarian cancer syndrome, hereditary non-polyposis colon cancer, or multiple endocrine neoplasia type 1. Direct sequencing of mutations is offered for the breast-ovarian cancer syndrome, for neurofibromatosis type 2, for multiple endocrine neoplasia type 2, and for families with features of the Li-Fraumeni syndrome (p53 analysis). If the particular test is not available in our laboratory, then the DNA is extracted locally and forwarded to a collaborator.

IV. FREQUENCY OF HEREDITARY CANCER

A cancer family is one in which there is sufficient evidence of the presence of a dominant cancer gene. Usually, this implies the presence of four or more cancers of a single site or of related sites (e.g., breast and ovary; colon and endometrium). Of the 411 cancer patients surveyed, 39 (9.5%) were judged to be members of cancer families. In comparison, only 3 of the 317 (0.9%) noncancer patients were judged to be members of cancer families. We do not know the actual proportion of eligible patients who completed and returned the questionnaire, and it is possible that members of cancer families were more likely to respond than isolated cancer cases.

The majority of cancer families were from recognized syndromes. However, approximately 40% of the probable cancer families were not identified as belonging to one of the classical dominant cancer syndromes (Table 1).

Of the 42 probands from cancer families, 29 underwent a complete genetic evaluation in the Division of Medical Genetics. The remaining 13 included 4 who were not possible to contact, and 2 who refused the offer of genetic counseling. The remaining seven cases are awaiting further evaluation. We found that by obtaining pedigree information by telephone we were able to

TABLE 1
Distribution of Hereditary Cancer Syndromes
Identified by Questionnaire

Syndrome	Number of families
Hereditary breast cancer	14
Hereditary breast-ovarian cancer	4
Familial melanoma	5
Hereditary non-polyposis colon cancer	5
Other/unknown syndromes	16
Total	42

decrease substantially the number of patients coming for genetic evaluation. Of 78 patients who received telephone calls, 24 were judged to be hereditary. Approximately three phone calls were made per hereditary case identified. The duration of the average phone call is approximately 20 minutes, whereas the genetic counseling session takes, on average, 1 hour.

V. CONCLUSION

In conclusion, we feel that it is reasonable to obtain a brief family history on all cancer patients through a self-administered questionnaire and to follow up on those with suggestive histories by telephone interview. By this method, we estimate that roughly 10% of McGill cancer patients are from cancer familes, but less than 1% of the general patient population at our hospital appears to be from cancer families.

Chapter 17

THE CATALOG OF HUMAN GENES PREDISPOSING TO NEOPLASIA

John J. Mulvihill, Sean Davis, Kenneth R. Fromkin

CONTENTS

I. INTRODUCTION

Throughout this volume, numerous single gene traits that predispose to malignancy are mentioned; however, it might be useful to consider the full range of genes and hereditary conditions that have been associated with neoplasia.

A tabulation in 1975[1] enumerated 161 mendelian traits that were associated with neoplasia, representing 9% of monogenic disorders known in 1971;[2] a 1977 update brought the number to 200;[3,4] in 1989, it was 338.[5,6]

For several years, the ongoing tally has been increasingly difficult to maintain, as the international human genome project to map and sequence all human genes has been launched and produced an avalanche of findings; in addition, the list of human protoncogenes, tumor suppressor genes, and mutator genes enlarges. McKusick published his eleventh edition in 1994,[7] and the entire database is updated daily as *Online Mendelian Inheritance in Man*. Nonetheless, we are in the midst of completing the genetic repertory of human neoplasia as it stands in late-1995,[8] and a preliminary tabulation is available (Table).

TABLE
Catalog of Human Preneoplastic Genes

Name	Inheritance[a]	Chromosome Location	Tumor Type
Alimentary System			
Anal canal carcinoma	AD	11q22-qter	Anal canal carcinoma
Barrett esophagus	AD		Esophageal adenocarcinoma
Blood group, Lewis system	AD*	19p13.1-q13	Gastrointestinal cancer
Carcinoid of intestine	AD		Multiple endocrine neoplasia
Cheilitis glandularis	AD		Squamous cell carcinoma, lower lip
Colorectal cancer-related chromosome sequence 17	AD*	17p12	Colorectal tumor
Colorectal cancer-related chromosome sequence 18	AD*	18q23.3	Colorectal tumor
Cystic fibrosis	AR*	7q31	Intestinal adenocarcinoma, especially of illeum
Focal epithelial hyperplasia of the oral mucosa	AD		Focal epithelial hyperplasia of the oral mucosa
Giant cell hepatitis, neonatal	AR*		Hepatic cancer
Hemangiomas of small intestine	AD		Hemangiomas of small intestine
Hemochromatosis	AR*	6p21.3	Hepatocellular carcinoma

Disorder	Inheritance	Location	Associated neoplasia
Hepatic adenomas, familial	AD		Sclerocystic ovaries; Hepatocellular carcinoma
Hepatocellular carcinoma 1	AD*	11p14-p13	Hepatocellular carcinoma
Hepatocellular carcinoma 2	AD*	4q32.1	Hepatocellular carcinoma
Leiomyoma of vulva and esophagus	AD		Leiomyoma of vulva; Leiomyoma of esophagus
Leukemia, acute myelocytic, with polyposis coli and colon cancer	AR		Leukemia, acute myelocytic; Colon cancer
Lip, hamartomatous	AD		Lip, hamartomatous
Lynch family cancer syndrome	AD*	18q11-q12	Colon cancer; Endometrium cancer; Ovarian cancer; Breast cancer
Lynch family cancer syndrome (MLH1)	AD*	3p21.3	Colon cancer; Endometrium cancer; Ovarian cancer; Breast cancer
Lynch family cancer syndrome (MSH2)	AD*	2p16-p15	Colon cancer; Endometrium cancer; Ovarian cancer; Breast cancer

TABLE (continued)
Catalog of Human Preneoplastic Genes

Name	Inheritance[a]	Chromosome Location	Tumor Type
Alimentary System (continued)			
Lynch family cancer syndrome (PMSL1)	AD*	2q31-q33	Colon cancer Endometrium cancer Ovarian cancer Breast cancer
Lynch family cancer syndrome (PMSL2)	AD*	7q22	Colon cancer Endometrium cancer Ovarian cancer Breast cancer
Methane production	AR*		Colon cancer
Milia, multiple eruptive	AD*		Colon carcinoma
Muir-Torre syndrome	AD*	2p16-p15	Cutaneous sebaceous neoplasms Keratocanthomas Gastrointestinal carcinomas Urogenital carcinomas
Oral facial digital syndrome type 3	AR*		Hamartoma, tongue
Oral facial digital syndrome type 4	AR		Tibial dysplasia Hamartoma, tongue

Condition	Inheritance	Locus	Tumor
Pancreatic carcinoma	AR		Pancreatic carcinoma
Pancreatitis, hereditary	AD*	5q22-q23	Pancreatic carcinoma
Polyposis, adenomatous intestinal	AD*		Colonic carcinoma
Polyposis coli, juvenile type	AD*		Colonic carcinoma
Polyposis, familial of entire gastrointestinal tract	AD		Colonic carcinoma
Polyposis, gastric	AD		Stomach adenocarcinoma
Polyposis, generalized juvenile with pulmonary arteriovenous malformaion	AD		Colon cancer
Polyposis, hamartomatous (Peutz-Jeghers)	AD*		Ovarian granulosa cell tumor Intestinal carcinoma Bilateral testicular tumor Pancreatic cancer
Polyposis, intestinal, scattered and discrete	AD		Gastric cancer Colon cancer
Polyposis, intestinal, with multiple exostoses	AD		Exostoses Sigmoid polyps Gastric polyps

TABLE (continued)
Catalog of Human Preneoplastic Genes

Name	Inheritance[a]	Chromosome Location	Tumor Type
Alimentary System (continued)			
Polyposis, skin pigmentation, alopecia, and fingernail changes	AD		Colon polyps
Porphyria cutanea tarda	AD*	1p34	Hepatocellular carcinoma
Turcot syndrome	AR*	5q21-22 7p22 3p21.3	Central nervous system tumors Colon polyposis
Tyrosinemia type 1	AR*		Postcirrhotic hepatoma
Cardiorespiratory System			
Acrocephalosyndactyly type 3 (Saethre-Chotzen)	AD*	7p21.3-p21.2	Nasopharyngeal carcinoma
Aryl hydrocarbon hydroxylase	AD		Bronchogenic carcinoma
Cancer of lung	AR		Cancer of lung
Fibrocystic pulmonary dysplasia	AD		Bronchial adenocarcinoma
Kartagener syndrome	AR*		Bronchogenic carcinoma

Mesothelioma, malignant	AD		Mesothelioma, malignant
Myxoma, intracardic	AR		Myxoma, intracardic
Nasopharyngeal cancer	AD		Nasopharyngeal cancer
Pulmonary alveolar proteinosis	AR*		Hematologic malignancies Lymphoma
Pulmonary fibrosis, idiopathic	AD		Alveolar cell carcinoma
Sarcoidosis	AD		Alveolar cell carcinoma
Scleroderma, familial progressive	AD		Alveolar cell carcinoma
Small cell cancer of the lung	AD		Small cell cancer of the lung
Ventricular hypertrophy, hereditary	AD		Ventricular hypertrophy

Chemical Markers

Alpha-fetoprotein	AD*	4q11-q13	Hepatocellular carcinoma Teratoma
Antitrypsin deficiency	AD*	14q32.1	Hepatocellular carcinoma
Calcitonin	AD*	11p15.4	Medullary thyroid carcinoma

TABLE (continued)
Catalog of Human Preneoplastic Genes

Name	Inheritance[a]	Chromosome Location	Tumor Type
Chemical Markers			
Chromogranin A	AD*	14q32	Pheochromocytoma Parathyroid adenoma Medullary thyroid carcinoma Carcinoid Oat-cell lung cancer Pancreatic islet cell tumor
Coagulation factor X deficiency	AR*	13q34	Carotid body tumor
Collagen type 6 alpha 1 chain	AD*	21q22.3	Multiple articular dysplasia Protuberant tumors
Cryoglobulinemia, familial mixed	AD*		Multiple myeloma
Cytochrome P450 family 2 subfamily D	AD*	22q11.2-q12	Lung cancer
Fucosidosis	AR*	1p34	Angiokeratoma
Gangliosidosis generalized GM1 type 3	AR	3p21.33	Angiokeratoma Spondyloepiphyseal dysplasia

Gastrin-releasing polypeptide	AD*	18q21	Pulmonary carcinoid Lung small cell carcinoma
Glutathione transferase 1	AD*	1p31	Lung cancer Hepatocellular carcinoma
Glycogen storage disease 1	AR*		Liver adenoma Hepatocellular carcinoma Hepatoblastoma
Glycogen storage disease 1B	AR*		Hepatic adenoma

Endocrine System

Acromegaly	AD		Pituitary tumor
Adrenal hyperplasia, 3	AR*	6p21.3	Gynecomastia Testicular tumor Sarcoma Astrocytoma
Adrenal hyperplasia, 5	AR*	10	Pulmonary liposarcoma
Adrenal hyperplasia, congenital	AR		Adrenal cortical tumor
Adrenocortical carcinoma, hereditary	AR		Adrenocortical carcinoma

TABLE (continued)
Catalog of Human Preneoplastic Genes

Name	Inheritance[a]	Chromosome Location	Tumor Type
Endocrine System (continued)			
Amenorrhea-galactorrhea syndrome	AD		Pituitary adenoma
Chemodectoma, intraabdominal, with cutaneous angiolipomas	AD		Chemodectoma / Cutaneous angiolipomas
Cushing disease, adrenal	AR		Adrenal cortical carcinoma
Dexamethasone-sensitive aldosteronism	AD*		Adrenal cortical adenoma
Familial cystic parathyroid adenomatosis	AD		Fibrous maxillary tumor / Fibrous mandibular tumor
Familial hypocalciuric hypercalcemia	AD*	3q21-q24	Lipomas
Familial primary hyperparathyroidism	AD*	11q13	Parathyroid adenoma / Chief cell hyperplasia
Goiter, nontoxic with intrathyroidal calcification	AD		Goiter
Hypoglycemia, leucine-induced	AR*		Islet cell adenoma

Hypophosphatemia, X-linked	XR*	Xp22	Parathyroid adenoma
Hypothalamic hamartoblastoma hypopituitarism	AD		Renal dysplasia Nail dysplasia
Macrosomia adiposa congenita	AR		Adrenocortical adenoma
Medullary thyroid carcinoma, familial	AD	10q21.1	Medullary thyroid carcinoma
Multiple endocrine neoplasia 1	AD*	11q13	Islet cell adenoma Parathyroid adenoma Pituitary adenoma Adrenal adenoma Malignant schwannoma Nonappendical carcinoid
Multiple endocrine neoplasia 2	AD*	10q21.1	Medullary thyroid carcinoma Parathyroid adenoma Pheochromocytoma
Multiple mucosal neuroma syndrome (multiple endocrine neoplasia 2b)	AD*	10q21.1	Pheochromocytoma Medullary thyroid carcinoma Neurofibroma Tongue submucosal neuroma Lip submucosal neuroma Eyelid submucosal neuroma
Nesidioblastosis of pancreas	AR*		Langerhans hyperplasia
Neuroblastoma	AR	1p36	Ganglioneuroma Pheochromocytoma

TABLE (continued)
Catalog of Human Preneoplastic Genes

Name	Inheritance[a]	Chromosome Location	Tumor Type
			Renal cell carcinoma
Endocrine System (continued)			
Nontoxic goiter with intrathyroidal calcification	AD*	8q24	Benign goiter
Paraganglioma	AD*	13q34	Pheochromocytoma Paraganglioma
Parathyroid adenomatosis, familial cystic	AD*		Jaw fibroma Parathyroid adenoma
Pheochromocytoma	AD*		Renal cell carcinoma Neuroblastoma
Pheochromocytoma, familial extraadrenal	AD		Pheochromocytoma
Pheochromocytoma–islet cell tumor syndrome	AD		Pheochromocytoma Islet cell tumor Islet cell carcinoma
Pineal hyperplasia insulin-resistant diabetes	AR*		Ovarian tumor Dental dysplasia

Pituitary dwarfism with large sella turcica	AR		Pituitary adenoma
Rothmund-Thomson syndrome	AR*		Paraganglioma Osteosarcoma
Thyroid carcinoma, papillary	AD	10q	Colon cancer Intraabdominal malignancies
Thyroid hormone, plasma membrane transport defect	AD		Goiter
Thyroid hormone resistance	AD*		Goiter
Thyroid hormonogenesis, genetic defect 2A	AR*	2pter-p12	Goiter
Thyroid hormonogenesis, genetic defect 2B	AR*	8q24	Goiter
Thyroid hormonogenesis, genetic defect 3	AR*		Goiter
Thyroid hormonogenesis, genetic defect 4	AR*		Goiter
Thyroid hormonogenesis, genetic defect 5	AR		Goiter
Thyrotoxic periodic paralysis	AD		Adrenal cortical adenoma
Thyrotoxicosis	AR		Goiter

Hemolymphatic System

Agranulocytosis infantile, genetic (Kostman)	AR*	6p21.3	Leukemia

TABLE (continued)
Catalog of Human Preneoplastic Genes

Name	Inheritance[a]	Chromosome Location	Tumor Type
Hemolymphatic System (continued)			
Anemia congenital hypoplastic (Blackfan-Diamond)	AR		Leukemia
DK phocomelia syndrome	AR		Myeloid leukemoid reaction
Eosinophilia, familial	AD		Collagenosis
Fanconi pancytopenia type 1	AR*	20q13.2-13.3	Acute myelogenous leukemia
Hodgkin disease	AR		Lymphocytic leukemia Lung adenocarcinoma
Incontinentia pigmenti	XD*	Xp11.2	Leukemia Retinoblastoma
Macroglobulinemia of Waldenstrom	AD		Lymphoma Lung adenocarcinoma Lymphocytic leukemia, chronic
Metaphyseal chondrodysplasia, McKusick	AR*		Lymphoma
Mycosis fungoides	AR		Hodgkin disease Leukemia

Disorder	Inheritance	Location	Neoplasm
Myeloma multiple	AR		Lymphoma; Multiple myeloma
Orthostatic hypotension	AD*		Plasmacytoma
Pelger-Huet anomaly	AD*		Burkitt lymphoma
Platelet disorder, undefined	AD		Acute lymphoblastic leukemia
Poland syndrome	AD		Neuroblastoma; Hematologic neoplasm
Polycythemia rubra vera	AR		Leukemia
Prader-Willi syndrome	AD*	15q11	Acute myelogenous leukemia; Leukemia
Reticuloendotheliosis, X-linked	XR*		Malignant reticuloendothelioma
Rubinstein syndrome	AR		Acute lymphoblastic leukemia
WT limb blood syndrome	AD		Leukemia

Immunodeficiency

Disorder	Inheritance	Location	Neoplasm
Agammaglobulinemia	XR*	Xq21.3-q22	Leukemia; Lymphoreticular neoplasia

TABLE (continued)
Catalog of Human Preneoplastic Genes

Name	Inheritance[a]	Chromosome Location	Tumor Type
Immunodeficiency (continued)			
Agammaglobulinemia, Swiss type	XR*	Xq13.1-q21.1	Leukemia Lymphoreticular neoplasia
Ataxia-telangiectasia	AR*	11q22-q23	Lymphoreticular neoplasia Leukemia Stomach carcinoma Brain tumors
Chediak Higashi-like syndrome	AR*		Pseudolymphoma
Immunodeficiency, X-linked progressive	XR*	Xq26	Ileum lymphoma Central nervous system lymphoma
Wiskott-Aldrich syndrome	XR*	Xp11.3-p11	Lymphoreticular neoplasia Leukemia
Multiple System			
Beckwith-Wiedemann (EMG) syndrome	AD*	11pter-p15.4	Visceromegaly Cytomegaly Macroglossia

Syndrome	Inheritance	Location	Neoplasms
			Adrenal cortical neoplasms Renal medullary blastoma Wilms tumor
Bloom syndrome	AR*	19q13.2-q13.3	Wilms tumor Esophageal cancer Intestinal cancer
Cancer, familial, with *in vitro* radioresistance	AD	17p13.1	Sarcoma, soft tissue Breast cancer Osteosarcoma Adrenal neoplasia Lung cancer Leukemia, acute
Cerebral gigantism (Sotos syndrome)	AD*	3p21	Hamartomatous intestinal polyps
Dyskeratosis congenita	XR*	Xq28	Squamous carcinoma Leukoplakia Hodgkin disease Pancreatic adenocarcinoma
Fanconi-like syndrome	AR		Cutaneous malignancies Lymph node metastases
Li-Fraumeni cancer family syndrome	AD*	17p13.1	Soft tissue sarcomas Bone sarcomas Brain neoplasms Leukemia Laryngeal neoplasms Lung neoplasms Adrenal cortical neoplasms

TABLE (continued)
Catalog of Human Preneoplastic Genes

Name	Inheritance[a]	Chromosome Location	Tumor Type
Multiple System (continued)			
Microcephaly with normal intelligence	AR*		Lymphoreticular malignancies Leukemia Generalized malignancies Hemoblastoma Lymphogranuloma Blastoma
SC phocomelia syndrome	AR		Hemangioma Hypoplastic cartilage Malignant melanoma
Nervous System			
Adaptin, beta, 1	AR*		Meningioma
AHNAK gene	AD*	11p13	Neuroblastoma
Amaurotic idiocy, adult type	AR		Astrocytoma
Blue rubber bleb nevus	AD*	9p	Cerebellar medulloblastoma Lymphocytic leukemia

Cerebral sarcoma	AD		Cerebral sarcoma
Chordoma	AR		Chordoma
Familial cavernous angioma	AD*	7q11-q22	Cerebral vascular angioma
Glioma of brain	AD		Bone cancer Muscle cancer Colonic polyps Skeletal exostoses
Hypothalamic hamartomas	AR		Glioma of brain
Macrocephaly multiple lipomas and hemangiomas	AD*		Intracranial tumors
Megalencephaly	AD		Ganglioneuroblastoma
Melanoma-astrocytoma syndrome	AD		Melanoma Astrocytoma
Meningioma	AD		Sarcoma, soft tissue Osteosarcoma Pinealoblastoma Melanoma, malignant
Myelocerebellar disorder	AD		Leukemia Bone marrow hypoplasia

TABLE (continued)
Catalog of Human Preneoplastic Genes

Name	Inheritance[a]	Chromosome Location	Tumor Type
Nervous System (continued)			
Neurofibromatosis 2	AD*	22q11.21-q13	Vestibular schwannomas Meningioma Schwannoma Neurofibroma
Neuronal ceroid lipofiscinosis	AD		Astrocytoma
Osteoporosis-pseudoglioma syndrome	AR		Glioma
Papilloma of choroid plexus	AR		Papilloma of choroid plexus
Pineal teratoma	AR		Medulloblastoma Paraventricular germinoma
Polysyndactyly with peculiar skull shape	AD*	7p13	Medulloblastoma
Pseudoglioma	AR		Glioma
Retinoblastoma	AD	13q14	Sarcoma Pinealoblastoma Melanoma
Seip syndrome	AR*		Hypothalamic glioma

Spinal extradural cyst	AR		Spinal extradural cyst
Transcobalamin II deficiency	AR		Meningioma
Usher syndrome	AR*		Metastatic cancer

Phacomatoses

Neurofibromatosis 1 (von Recklinghausen)	AD*	17q11.2	Fibrosarcoma Neurofibroma Schwannoma Meningioma Optic pathway glioma Pheochromocytoma
Proteus syndrome	AD	3p25-p24	Lipomatosis Conjunctival dermoid
Tuberous sclerosis	AD*	9q33-q34 16p13.3	Angiofibroma Periungual fibroma Glial tumors Rhabdomyoma of heart Renal tumor Lung cysts
von Hippel-Lindau disease	AD*	3p25-p24	Retinal angioma Cerebellar hemangioblastoma Hemangioma Pheochromocytoma Renal cell carcinoma Cysts

TABLE (continued)
Catalog of Human Preneoplastic Genes

Name	Inheritance[a]	Chromosome Location	Tumor Type
Skeletal System			
Cherubism	AD		Jaw fibrous dysplasia Giant cell tumor
Chondrosarcoma	AR		Chondrosarcoma
Dysplasia epiphysealis hemimelica with chondromas	AD*		Chondromas Osteochondromas
Enchondromatosis, generalized	AR		Enchondromatosis
Exostoses, multiple	AD*	8q23-q24.1	Osteosarcoma Chondrosarcoma
Exostoses of external auditory canal	AD		Ear exostoses
Exostoses of heel	AD		Exostoses
Exostoses with anetodermia and brachydactyly, type E	AD		Exostoses
Frontofacionasal dysostosis	AR*		Limbic dermoid Lipomata

Genochondromatosis	AD		Chondromatosis
Metachondromatosis	AD		Chondromatosis
Multiple exostoses with spastic tetraparesis	AD		Exostoses
OSLAM syndrome	AD		Osteosarcoma
Osteochondromatosis	AD		Chondrosarcoma Ovarian juvenile granulosa cell tumor
Osteosarcoma	AR		Osteosarcoma
Paget disease of bone	AD	6p21.3	Osteosarcoma
Polyostotic fibrous dysplasia	AD		Hyperthyroidism
Ramon syndrome	AR		Maxillary fibrous dysplasia Gingival fibromatosis
Spondylometaphyseal dysplasia with enchondromatous changes	AR		Enchondromatosis
Upington disease	AD*		Endochondroma

Skin and Its Appendages

Albinism 1 (occulocutaneous)	AR*	11q14-q21	Melanoma Skin cancers

TABLE (continued)
Catalog of Human Preneoplastic Genes

Name	Inheritance[a]	Chromosome Location	Tumor Type
Skin and Its Appendages (continued)			
Albinism with hemorrhagic diathesis	AR*		Pulmonary fibrosis Cutaneous malignant melanoma
Bazex syndrome	AD		Basal cell carcinoma
Cardiomyopathy hypogonadism collagenoma syndrome	AD		Cutaneous collagenoma
Cerumen, variation in	AD		Breast cancer
Charcot-Marie-Tooth disease	AD*	1q22-q23	Malignant melanoma
Dysplastic nevus syndrome, hereditary (CMM1)	AD*	1p36	Cutaneous malignant melanoma Colon cancer
Dysplastic nevus syndrome, hereditary (CMM2)	AD*	9p13-p22	Cutaneous malignant melanoma Colon cancer Pancreatic cancer
Epidermodysplasia verruciformis	AR		Squamous cell carcinoma, skin

Epidermodysplasia verruciformis, X-linked	XR		Squamous cell carcinoma, skin
Epidermolysis bullosa dystrophica	AD*	12q11-q13	Squamous cell carcinoma, skin
Epithelioma hereditary multiple benign cystic	AD*		Basosquamous cell carcinoma Spiradenoma
Fibrofolliculomas with trichodiscomas	AD		Trichodiscomas Acrochordons
Hyperkeratosis lenticularis perstans	AD*		Skin tumors
Ichthyosis, X-linked	XR*	Xpter-p22.32	Seminoma
Keratosis palmoplantaris with periodontopathia	AR*		Apocrine hydrocystoma
Langer-Giedion syndrome	AD	8q24.11-q24	Multiple exostoses
Lichen planus, familial	AD		Oral carcinoma
Lichen sclerosus et atrophicus	AD		Squamous cell carcinoma, vulva
Lipomatosis, multiple	AD*	12q13-q14	Skin cancer
Melanoma, malignant intraocular	AD		Malignant intraocular melanoma
Melanoma, uveal	AD		Uveal melanoma
Melanosis neurocutaneous	AR		Malignant melanoma, skin Malignant melanoma, meninges

TABLE (continued)
Catalog of Human Preneoplastic Genes

Name	Inheritance[a]	Chromosome Location	Tumor Type
Skin and its Appendages (continued)			
Myxoma spotty pigmentaion and endocrine cancer (Carney) syndrome (NAME and LAMB syndromes)	AD*	2p16	Nevi Atrial myxoma Myxoid neurofibromas Fibromas Hemangiomas Adrenocortical carcinoma Papillary thyroid carcinoma Sertoli cell tumor
Nail-patella syndrome	AD*	9q34	Colon cancer
Pachynychia congenita, Jackson-Lawler type	AD		Oral leukokeratosis Cylindromas
Piebald trait	AD*	4q12	Epitheliomas
Porokeratosis of Mibelli	AD*		Skin cancer Colon adenocarcinoma
Roberts syndrome	AR*		Melanoma

	Inheritance	Location	Neoplasia
Rombo syndrome	AD		Trichoepitheliomas Basal cell carcinoma
Scleroatrophic and keratotic dermatosis of limbs	AD*	4q28-q31	Skin cancer Bowel cancer
Spiegler-Brooke tumors	XR		Epithelioma Cylindroma
Tooth and nail syndrome	AD*		Polycystic ovaries
Torticollis, keloids, cryptorchidism	XR*	Xq28	Basal cell epithelioma
Xeroderma pigmentosum	AR		Multiple skin cancer Melanoma Basal cell carcinoma
Xeroderma pigmentosum 1	AR*	9q34.2	Skin cancer
Xeroderma pigmentosum 2	AR*	2q21	Skin cancer
Xeroderma pigmentosum 3	AR*	3p25	Skin cancer Malignant melanoma
Xeroderma pigmentosum 4	AR*		Skin cancer
Xeroderma pigmentosum 5	AR*		Skin cancer
Xeroderma pigmentosum 6	AR*	15	Skin cancer

TABLE (continued)
Catalog of Human Preneoplastic Genes

Name	Inheritance[a]	Chromosome Location	Tumor Type
Skin and Its Appendages (continued)			
Xeroderma pigmentosum 7	AR*		Skin cancer
Xeroderma pigmentosum 9	AR		Skin cancer
Xeroderma pigmentosum with normal DNA repair rate	AR		Skin cancer
Xerodermic idiocy of De Sanctis and Cacchione	AR		Skin cancer
			Acute lymphocytic leukemia
Soft Tissues			
Adiposis dolorosa	AD		Subcutaneous lipomas
Branchial clefts with characteristic facies	AD		Hemangiomatous branchial cysts
Cowden multiple hamartoma syndrome	AD*		Papilloma, lip
			Papilloma, mouth
			Hypertrophic breast
			Cystic breast

Condition	Inheritance	Map	Neoplasia
			Thyroid adenoma / Thyroid carcinoma / Colon carcinoma / Colon adenoma and polyps
Fibromatosis, congenital generalized	AR		Multiple fibroblastic tumors
Fibromatosis, gingival with abnormal fingers, nails	AD*		Splenomegaly / Hepatomegaly
Fibromatosis, juvenile hyaline	AR*		Multiple subcutaneous tumors / Gingival fibromatosis
Lymphedema with distichiasis	AD*		Lymphangiosarcoma
Nevoid cell carcinoma syndrome	AD*	9q31	Basal cell carcinoma / Medulloblastoma / Jaw cysts / Ovarian fibroma and carcinoma
Werner syndrome	AR*	8p12-p11	Sarcoma

Urogenital System

Condition	Inheritance	Map	Neoplasia
Arrhenoblastoma—thyroid adenoma	AD		Arrhenoblastoma / Thyroid adenoma
Bladder cancer	AD		Bladder cancer
Cryptophthalmos with other malformations	AR*		Gonadoblastoma

TABLE (continued)
Catalog of Human Preneoplastic Genes

Name	Inheritance[a]	Chromosome Location	Tumor Type
Urogenital System (continued)			
Fraser syndrome	AD		Gonadoblastoma
Gestational trophoblastic disease	AR		Gestational trophoblastic disease
Gonadal dysgenesis, XY female type	XR*	Xp22-p21	Gonadoblastoma Germinoma
Gonadal dysgenesis, XY type	AR		Gonadal tumors
Hyperprolinemia type 1	AR*		Wilms tumor
Multiple hereditary leiomyomata of skin	AD*	18p11.32	Uterine myomas Myofibroma
Nephrosis, congenital	AR*		Wilms tumor
Ovarian fibromas	AD		Ovarian fibromata
Ovarian teratoma	AD		Ovarian teratoma
Ovarian tumor	AD*		Colon cancer

Disorder	Inheritance	Location	Manifestations
Perlman syndrome	AR*		Breast cancer Intraabdominal malignancies
Presacral teratoma with sacral dysgenesis	AD*		Renal hamartomas Nephroblastomatosis Wilms tumor
Renal cell carcinoma	AD		Medulloepithelial cancer
Stein-Leventhal syndrome	AD		Renal cell carcinoma
Systemic cystic angiomatous and Seip syndrome	AR		Ovarian cysts
Testicular tumors	AR*		Polycystic ovarian dysplasia
Ureter, cancer of	AD		Testicular tumors
Wilms tumor	AD*	11p13	Ureter, cancer of Gonadoblastoma
Wilms tumor and pseudohermaphroditism	AD		Wilms tumor

a A "*" next to the inheritance code denotes that McKusick feels the inheritance pattern has been verified.

II. THE PRELIMINARY TABLE

The table was prepared by cover-to-cover reading of the eighth edition of *Mendelian Inheritance in Man*[6] and an ongoing monitoring of the additions and deletions in subsequent editions, supplemented by online searches and reading of original journals. As of the 1994 edition,[7] there were 6678 entries of proven single gene traits or with suggestive but inconclusive evidence of mendelian behavior. In September 1995, simple word search produced 609 entries with the word *tumor*, 437 with *cancer*, 268 with *carcinoma*, and 218 with *neoplasia*, but much overlap surely occurs. Preliminary tally shows 467 (7%) entries that predispose or are associated with neoplasia (Table). The included traits are sometimes clinical phenotypes, diseases, or conditions, and sometimes proteins or DNA sequences of uncertain function. The 105 protoncogenes and 78 tumor suppressor genes have been omitted for reasons of space. A phenotype entry has been included when benign or malignant neoplasia or tumor occurs as a sole feature, a frequent concomitant, or just a rare complication of the trait. Because of their rarity, some disorders are represented by only single case reports. Certain entities may be contestable and others may be missing, e.g., not all known reports of familial aggregation of neoplasms of the same or diverse cell types are included.

Initially, the table was handled strictly as a word processing task. It seemed obvious that improved flexibility for searching and organization could be gained by maintaining a database of the same information. The current version, not yet complete, is maintained as a *Filemaker Pro* database on a Macintosh computer. The eight data fields currently included in the database are the name of condition or trait, the corresponding *Mendelian Inheritance in Man* code number, inheritance pattern, whether or not a gene has been isolated, chromosome localization (if known), the main organ system affected, associated neoplasia, and International Classification of Diseases (ICD) coding.

Sorting by various fields emphasizes differing aspects of the information. For example, a sort by chromosome localization reveals mapping information. Current sorting by tumor type is imperfect because of the different terminology that is used from entry to entry to describe similar neoplasms; nonetheless it is easy to spot six traits associated with breast tumors. A more revelant organization by tumor type awaits nosologic coding according to *The International Classification of Diseases*[9] and, where possible, specific coding by site and type of cancer.[10] The current presentation — admittedly somewhat arbitrary — is by organ system, not strictly of the major features of the trait, but rather by the organ system of the associated neoplasia. Hence, cystic fibrosis is NOT grouped under the respiratory tract, its major site of morbidity and mortality, but rather under alimentary tract, because the major associated neoplasm is adenocarcinoma of the small intestine.

III. LESSONS FROM THE TABLE

A. BIOLOGY OF CANCER

One of several points to be made from the Table is its length; a substantial portion of all known single gene traits in human beings is associated with neoplasia. In many, neoplasia is only an occasional feature that may arise at various ages; therefore, other factors in the environment or other genes must be interacting to produce tumor. Elsewhere is a list of 22 genetic traits that result in cancer with exposure to a specific environmental agent.[11]

Second, the table is the mutant genetic repertory of neoplasia in human beings. It emphasizes the large number of genes that might be involved in susceptibility to cancer, and, by inference, the number of normal genes that contribute to resistance to neoplasia. About 59% of the traits are autosomal dominant, passed on to about one-half of an affected person's offspring; 36% are autosomal recessive, requiring two mutant alleles to be manifested and more likely to occur in offspring of consanguineous couples; and 5% are X-linked traits, seen exclusively or more severely in males than females.

Third, nearly all histologic types of tumors are represented, including the commonest malignancies, those of the skin, breast, colon, and lung. These and other tumors occurring in monogenic traits are often morphologically indistinguishable from sporadically occurring tumors. Lung cancers of various types, for example, have been reported in antecedent pulmonary disorders that are sometimes familial (and probably genetic), in familial cancer syndromes, and in association with genetic biochemical markers. In these three categories, examples include, respectively, dominant fibrocystic pulmonary dysplasia and idiopathic pulmonary fibrosis and recessive cystic disease of the lung, sarcoidosis, and Kartagener syndrome; site-specific familial lung cancer and mesothelioma and the Li-Fraumeni (SBLA) cancer family syndrome; and, aryl hydrocarbon hydroxylase inducibility, a cytochrome P-450, and gastrin-releasing polypeptide. In short, histologic type is not a reliable flag for a neoplasm of single gene origin. Rather, mendelian traits associated with neoplasia may be identified by recognizing other features of the trait or syndrome in the patient or in family members.

Of the 284 preneoplastic gene traits given in the table, 83 (29%) have been mapped to a chromosomal band or at least assigned to a specific chromosome. Genes on every chromosome except 16 have been associated with a possibly increased risk of neoplasia. 79% of preneoplastic genes on chromosome X have been mapped, a high frequency of success attributable to the large number of available markers. 33% of the autosomal dominant and 16% of the autosomal recessive traits have been mapped; progress in mapping autosomal genes will increase as the international genome project produces increasingly dense genetic marker maps.

B. CLINICAL AND EPIDEMIOLOGIC APPLICATIONS

The clinician who diagnoses a person's cancer but not the syndrome of which it is a manifestation makes an incomplete diagnosis. Every surgeon who has a patient with breast cancer should look for small papillomas of the lips, gums, and palpebral fissures or hyperkeratotic papules of the hands, which would suggest the Cowden multiple hamartoma syndrome. Failure to recognize a rare syndrome is a disservice to the patient and perhaps relatives, who may be denied the possible benefits of counseling for prevention and early detection of cancer. Also, an opportunity for further research into pathogenesis is lost. Some of these traits were discovered because an unusual aggregation of cancer was seen and investigated in a family. In theory, any one of the traits could explain a cancer family.

The epidemiologist investigating cancer etiology, perhaps with a case-control study design, must be aware that histopathologically identical tumors may have different etiologies. Geneticists have long recognized the phenomenon of genetic heterogeneity, namely the fact that one phenotype (like shortness of stature and organomegaly) can be attributed to a number of different causes and, specifically, to various gene mutations. Pheochromocytoma can be a feature of neurofibromatosis 1, von Hippel-Lindau syndrome, multiple endocrine neoplasia types 2a and 2b (the Sipple syndrome and the multiple mucosal neuroma syndrome, respectively), multiple mucosal neuroma syndrome, and familial paraganglioma. Sarcomas of various types have been described in association with neurofibromatosis 1, retinoblastoma, congenital adrenal hyperplasia, meningioma, lymphedema with disichiasis, Paget disease of bone, multiple exostosis, OSLAM syndrome, osteochondromatosis, the Li-Fraumeni (SBLA) cancer family syndrome, familial cancer with *in vitro* radioresistance, Rothmund-Thomson syndrome, and Werner syndrome.

The epidemiologist concerned with cancer control might guess that the conditions in the table probably account for a small fraction of human cancer. A few, such as the intestinal polyposes, dysplastic nevus syndrome, and the breast cancer genes (*BRCA1* and *BRCA2*), clearly have public health implications. When these dominant traits are discovered in a patient, an opportunity arises to identify individuals at enormous risk for cancer. Such high risk persons are likely to be especially motivated to understanding and comply with a personalized prescription for cancer surveillance. As set forth by a NIH workshop,[12,13] it is reasonable to suggest that the clinical geneticist assume responsibility for alerting families to the hereditary and familial nature of the disorders that predispose to cancer and offering surveillance. Research in cancer prevention is best piloted in such individuals at highest risk by strict protocols involving intensive counseling and informed consent, especially when laboratory testing for major predisposing genes is planned. The broader significance is the possibility that intense study of these conditions may give insight into the etiology and pathogenesis of cancers in general.

ACKNOWLEDGMENTS

We thank Victor A. McKusick for his enduring support of our efforts to use his valuable catalogues for understanding human cancer genetics. A number of research assistants have helped over the years, including Wanda M. Wade, Patricia Madigan, Tammy Molinaro, Patricia Szymanski, Anita M. Socci, and Rana Snipe.

REFERENCES

1. **Mulvihill, J. J.,** Congenital and genetic diseases, Fraumeni, J. F., Jr., Ed., *Persons at High Risk of Cancer: An Approach to Cancer Etiology and Control*, Academic Press, New York, 1975, 3.
2. **McKusick, V. A.,** *Mendelian Inheritance in Man. Catalogs of Autosomal Dominant. Autosomal Recessive, and X-linked Phenotypes.* 3rd ed., The Johns Hopkins University Press, Baltimore, 1971, ix.
3. **Mulvihill, J. J.,** Genetic repertory of human neoplasia, in Mulvihill, J. J., Miller, R. W., and Fraumeni, J. F., Jr., Eds., *Genetics of Human Cancer*, Raven Press, New York, 1977, 137.
4. **McKusick, V. A.,** *Mendelian Inheritance in Man. Catalogs of Autosomal Dominant. Autosomal Recessive, and X-linked Phenotypes.* 4th ed., The Johns Hopkins University Press, Baltimore, 1974, xii.
5. **Mulvihill, J. J.,** Prospects for cancer control and prevention through genetics, *Clin. Genet.,* 36, 313–319, 1989.
6. **McKusick, V. A.,** *Mendelian Inheritance in Man. Catalogs of Autosomal Dominant. Autosomal Recessive, and X-linked Phenotypes.* 8th ed., The Johns Hopkins University Press, Baltimore, 1988, xi.
7. **McKusick, V. A.,** *Mendelian Inheritance in Man. A Catalog of Human Genes and Genetic Disorders.* 11th ed., The Johns Hopkins University Press, Baltimore, 1994, vii.
8. **Mulvihill, J. J.,** *McKusick's Mendelian Inheritance in Man for Oncology.* The Johns Hopkins University Press, Baltimore, 1996 (in press).
9. **U.S. Department of Health and Human Services, Public Health Service, Health Care Financing Administration**, *The International Classification of Diseases*, 9th ed., U.S. Government Publishing Office, Washington, D.C., 1991.
10. **Percy, C., Van Holten, V., and Muir, C., Eds.,** *International Classification of Diseases for Oncology*, World Health Organization, Geneva, 1990.
11. **Mulvihill, J. J.,** Clinical ecogenetics of human cancer, *Hem./Onc. Ann.*, 2, 157–161, 1994.
12. **Parry, D. M., Berg, K., Mulvihill, J. J., Carter, C. L., and Miller, R. W.,** Strategies for controlling cancer through genetics: Report of a workshop, *Am. J. Hum. Genet.*, 41, 63-69, 1987.
13. **Parry, D. M., Mulvihill, J. J., Miller, R. W., Berg, K., and Carter, C. C.,** Strategies for controlling cancer through genetics, *Cancer Res.*, 47, 6814-6817, 1987.

INDEX